IMAGES
of America

LONG ISLAND
STATE HOSPITALS

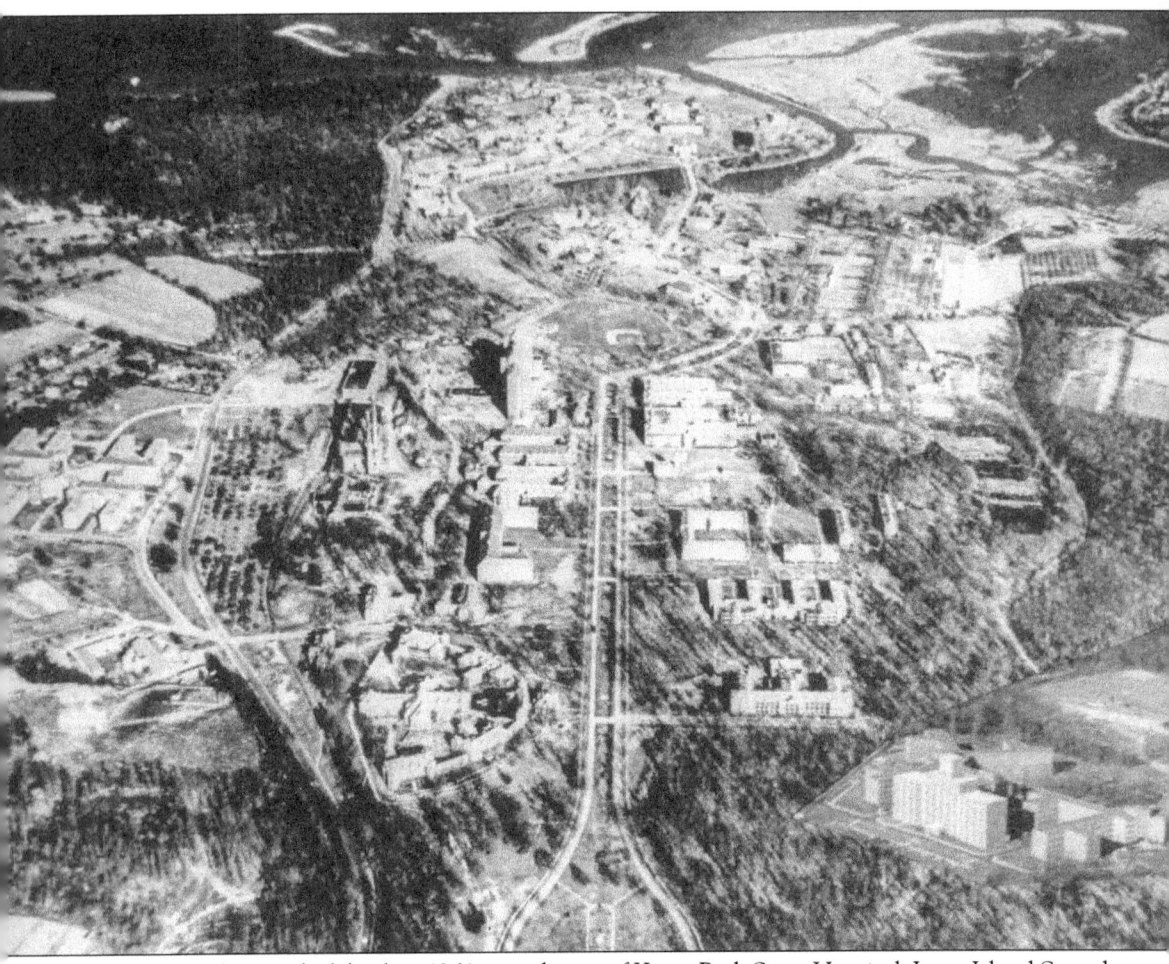

In the background of this late 1960s aerial view of Kings Park State Hospital, Long Island Sound is visible. At the time this picture was taken, the hospital had been in large scale operation, with over 100 buildings on the property. In the right foreground is the newly constructed medical/surgical services Building 7, which was erected to replace the older medical/surgical building located across the campus.

ON THE COVER: Men in three-piece suits and ties craft woven baskets at Kings Park State Hospital around 1900. This is a fantastic illustration of the attention to dignity and craftmanship at the hospital. The men enjoy a scenic view of the grounds and fresh air while engaged in activity. (Courtesy of the Kings Park Heritage Museum)

IMAGES of America
LONG ISLAND STATE HOSPITALS

Joseph M. Galante

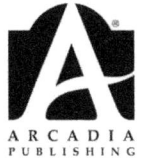

Copyright © 2019 by Joseph M. Galante
ISBN 978-1-4671-0358-9

Published by Arcadia Publishing
Charleston, South Carolina

Library of Congress Control Number: 2019941206

For all general information, please contact Arcadia Publishing:
Telephone 843-853-2070
Fax 843-853-0044
E-mail sales@arcadiapublishing.com
For customer service and orders:
Toll-Free 1-888-313-2665

Visit us on the Internet at www.arcadiapublishing.com

The book is dedicated to the memory of all the staff and patients at Central Islip, Kings Park, and Pilgrim State Hospitals.

Contents

Acknowledgments		6
Introduction		7
1.	From Farm Colonies to Hospitals	11
2.	Nursing and Medical Staff	33
3.	Fire, Police, and Wartime	51
4.	The Farms and Shops	67
5.	Life and Activities on the Grounds	79

ACKNOWLEDGMENTS

This publication was substantially inspired by the author's personal experience in working with, befriending, and admiring many tremendous staff and patients who were a part of the Long Island state hospitals' legacy. The book would not have been possible without the expansive amount of time and energy from individuals who shared photographs and their most intimate experiences, resulting from decades of service in public mental healthcare.

    I was afforded an eye-opening internship opportunity during the spring of my freshman year in college at a public psychiatric institution. The time spent under the tutelage of the outgoing generation of hospital staff, who lived the changes in public behavioral health firsthand, for better and worse, was invaluable. Words cannot express my thanks to all the women and men I was privileged to work with in public service for impacting my life and career in unimaginable ways. I offer my extraordinary gratitude to the following people for their guidance, encouragement, and willingness to help me mature as a person and professional: Alfred "Al" Cibelli, Vivian Dellera, Jaclyn "Jackie" Vercellone, "Nan" Nancy Steen, Elena Geonie, James "Jimmy" Kilkenny, Elizabeth "Betty" Macchia, Nina Lomangino, Diana Dantuono, and Donna Crook. A very special thank-you to John Leita and his wife, Laura Cummings, for sharing their time, knowledge, and resources to compile the material for this book. I express much gratitude to a colleague and friend, Craig Williams, retired senior historian at the New York State Museum, for his wisdom, personal time, and curatorial expertise. For her historical and technical sagacity, I extend my appreciation to my confidant, co-curator, and co-author of *The Hudson River State Hospital*, Lynn Rightmyer, RN. Lastly, I thank my friends and family, especially my mother and father, for their backing and cheering to finalize this production. Unless otherwise noted, all images appear courtesy of a private collection.

INTRODUCTION

New York City was a bustling and rapidly expanding place of industry and immigration in the 1800s. Steamships made the voyage across the Atlantic Ocean faster than ever. As a result, the number of immigrants coming to America in search of work and a new life increased. With the growth of the nation came a greater number of mentally ill individuals requiring psychiatric hospitalization. Existing facilities to treat the mentally ill at the New York City asylums were becoming overtaxed; overcrowding and understaffing grew worse yearly. To alleviate overcrowding at the Kings County Lunatic Asylum in Flatbush, plans were made to purchase land and construct a sister facility to the east in Suffolk County in 1884. The board of supervisors at the Kings County Asylum were authorized to procure "a site at St. Johnland . . . for the purpose of providing increased accommodations for paupers, the insane, and other county wards." Accomplishments of the Society of St. Johnland, an orphanage and home for the disabled and poor of New York City, had caught the attention of the Kings County Asylum administration. In 1885, the state assembly sanctioned the purchase of approximately 850 acres at St. Johnland to alleviate the overcrowding at Kings County and start a "branch asylum." By the fall of that year, 23 women and 33 men were transferred to the branch asylum into three temporary wooden buildings.

Dr. John C. Shore, superintendent of the Kings County Asylum, was charged with establishing and supervising the new branch asylum at St. Johnland. The plans were to erect buildings on a cottage model consisting of 16 wood-frame wards for 450 patients. Additionally, a laundry facility, heating plant, several barns, and other ancillary buildings were to be constructed. Progress was slow, as the first two permanent cottages were not opened until June 18, 1888, lacking heat and only providing a limited supply of water. The remainder of the cottages were constructed over the coming year and were filled beyond capacity almost immediately. Ironically, due to the soaring number of insane in New York City, the overcrowding was actually worse at the Kings County Asylum than ever before. Continual admissions to the asylum led to the planning and development of four additional brick buildings to accommodate 600 patients and 14 more cottages at the branch for a total of 34 patient buildings by 1892. Roads were graded, sewers were installed, electric light and steam heating systems were operational, a laundry was opened, and a bakery was functioning as well by the end of the year.

The facility was receiving and treating over 1,000 patients per year and was regarded largely as a success, despite abandoning its original intent of alleviating overcrowding at Flatbush. The principal psychiatric treatment was moral therapy, which had gained serious traction as a result of Quaker physician Thomas Story Kirkbride's work in the mid-19th century. Patients were encouraged to spend time on the hospital grounds, work, sew, and engage in art and music as they labored toward recovery, with an ultimate goal of restoration to society. The environment in which care was delivered was viewed as being equally important to the therapy itself. This unity of Quaker religious values and science was largely successful in the healing of the symptoms that ailed many patients.

Programs aimed at the care and rehabilitation of patients kept pace with the facility's growth until 1890. A new administration of the Kings County Board of Charities and Corrections, which oversaw both the Kings County Asylum and the St. Johnland branch, described the previous standards of moral therapy to be "completely out of tune with the purpose" of operating. The new administrators stopped the patients from farming, a cornerstone of their therapy, on the impression that produce procured from markets would be more cost-effective. Trained attendants were dismissed from employment and replaced by staff hired through political favors. The newly successful county farm was becoming disappointingly idle and stagnant. Disheartened by the changes, and reaching an elder age, Supt. Dr. John Macumber resigned in 1892. He was replaced by a younger, more spirited physician, Dr. Oliver M Dewing. Under Superintendent Dewing's tenure, the facility was on a path back toward the county farm's original success. However, this was not without hindrances. With the new county administration in 1890 came new construction on the grounds of the branch asylum. Contractors were chosen based on political patronage and bribes. A cow barn was constructed for $80,000, which should have not cost more than $12,000. A barge carrying cement to grade a road sprung a leak on the way to the county farm. Hundreds of barrels of useless cement were paid for and described as being in good condition upon arrival. Hundreds of wagonloads of dirt were hauled off to a wooded site after trenching out a water reservoir, only to be returned to build an embankment around it. A committee of the state assembly was formed to investigate the affairs of the Kings County Asylum at Flatbush and St. Johnland. It was remarked at the conclusion of the investigation,

> From almost the beginning of the administration of the Department by Commissioners Gott, Nolan and Murphy, in 1890, their purpose in violating the Statute is indicated by the removal of subordinates of acknowledged capacity and honesty. Their places were filled by men of no expertise in respect to the duties to be performed, or if not deficient in capacity, of doubtful integrity. . . . I may say generally that the standard of care and treatment of the Insane in Kings County was, and had been for years previous to that, very, very much below that of any other locality in the State.

The findings of the committee were in accord with the prevailing public sentiment, calling for the removal of Kings County's custodianship over the Brooklyn and St. Johnland sites. Despite the county's vehement opposition, fraud and flagrant financial mismanagement by the Kings County administration led to the asylum's transfer of ownership and operation to the State of New York in 1895. No longer was the primary purpose of the branch asylum to alleviate overcrowding in Brooklyn. Hope for positive reform both in Brooklyn and the newly renamed Long Island State Hospital at Kings Park (later renamed Kings Park State Hospital) under the state's control came to be a reality. Nine hundred patients were transferred from the Manhattan State Hospital to a new group of buildings at Kings Park that same year. The growth of Kings Park now seemed unstoppable, soon becoming a site more critical to state operations than the mother hospital in Brooklyn. Kings Park was administered from afar at Brooklyn until May 1, 1900, when it was officially declared to be a separate state hospital.

Eleven miles southeast of Kings Park in a village of few houses, two stores, and one post office, another farm colony was established. Central Islip began receiving patients in 1888 from the City of New York. The colony paralleled Kings Park, opening with the intention of alleviating overcrowding at city asylums. Specifically, the New York City Asylum for the Insane divisions on Ward, Blackwell, and Hart Islands were to be affected. Purchased in 1887 and located 45 miles east of New York City, the colony was reached by a one-track branch line off the main line of the Long Island Rail Road. The colony at Central Islip was established with the purpose to "promote rational outdoor living, exercise, and occupation" in a tranquil location, distinctly different than the overcrowded city streets of Manhattan where many of the patients came from. The colony was opened as an experiment under the supervision of the New York City Board of Charities and Corrections and administered from Manhattan. The experimental farm colony was positioned to examine the progress of chronically ill patients and improvements in their quality of life over a period of three years. Three groups of three wards—A, B, and C—were raised in wood frame buildings and arranged with a dining room, small bakery, and attached kitchen to support and house the first patients. In the spring of 1889, the first year, 140 male patients arrived. That summer, they cleared 15 to 20 acres of pine and oak scrub for use as farmland and successfully planted grain. The Board of Charities and Corrections for the City of New York promised the replacement of the wood frame buildings with permanent brick structures at the close of the farm colony experiment if it proved a success. However, they were not demolished until February 1940.

The farm colony was remarkably successful by the close of the three-year evaluation period in 1892. The city asylums transferred 40 women from both Blackwell and Hart Islands to Ward A-1 to aid with the laundry service. Previously, clothes and linens had been transported by rail to New York City for laundering. By 1893, contracts were procured to build three more groups—D, E, and F—out of brick on a one-story plan to the northeast of the main grounds. Currently, one of these buildings remains as the Recreation Center for the Town of Central Islip. Similar to the initial structures, each group consisted of three detached wards with a dining room. By 1894, approximately 300 patients occupied nine buildings, supervised by two physicians who made rounds, instructed nursing staff, treated patients, directed grounds squads, and administered the colony. By 1895, Dr. George A. Smith was appointed the first superintendent of the Farm Colony at Central Islip. He was instrumental in guiding the facility onto a more progressive track. Dr. Smith had transferred to Central Islip from his position at Hart Island as superintendent of the New York City Asylum. That same year, 700 additional patients were also transferred from both Ward and Hart Island. The patient census by the close of 1895 was over 1,000 men and women. At the time, the colony had 30 buildings, a farm, roads, gardens, and lawns, and was noted for its grand appearance.

On February 2, 1896, the New York City Asylums for the Insane were transferred to the state, including the colony at Central Islip. Now falling under the umbrella of Manhattan State Hospital, the city facilities had four divisions: Manhattan State Hospital East for Men, Manhattan State West for Women (both on Wards Island), Manhattan State for both sexes on Hart Island (decommissioned in 1898), and Manhattan State Hospital at Central Islip for both sexes. In 1899, Central Islip had six physicians, 154 male and 44 female employees, and 1,074 patients, of which 744 were male. By June 1905, the newly christened Central Islip State Hospital became its own separate, independent facility.

Largely due to provisions of the State Care Act of 1890, for the remainder of their time as functioning psychiatric hospitals, Kings Park and Central Islip flourished under state control. The Long Island state hospitals' populations continued to expand into the 20th century. By the 1920s, the need for another facility had become apparent. During New York's 1925 constitutional reorganization, the state Department of Mental Hygiene was created, with the purpose of mental health management, logistics, and oversight of public institutional care. Pilgrim State Hospital was commissioned by the legislature in 1926 as a "final solution" to alleviate the overcrowding at the four state institutions caring for New York City's mentally ill: Brooklyn, Central Islip, Kings Park, and Manhattan State Hospital. Gov. Alfred E. Smith was a well-known and longtime advocate for both the state's mentally ill and hospital facilities. He was chiefly responsible, through his personal urging of the legislature, for the securing of $50 million to construct a new facility. A large facility of similar proportions was under construction at the same time in Rockland County, just above the city. The Department of Mental Hygiene's planning board had agreed that approximately 1,000 acres would be sufficient to build the hospital. Acquiring that amount of land in the city was impractical. The site would need access from rail and highway, have appropriate space to farm, and a water supply and sewage disposal. After consideration of needs, Long Island once again fit the board's requirements. A site in Suffolk County near Brentwood was owned by one person and eligible for sale at an affordable price. On April 20, 1928, Dr. Parsons, commissioner of the Department of Mental Hygiene, authorized the purchase of 1,056.8 acres of land for the price of $308,800. A sum of $1 million was made accessible immediately for the new state hospital to procure construction contracts. Male wards Building 1 and Building 2, along with Kitchen 3, were among the first buildings constructed in 1929. Gov. Franklin D. Roosevelt signed the bill naming Pilgrim State Hospital on April 10, 1929. Pilgrim was designed to accommodate 10,000 patients on an urban campus named after the revered commissioner of the Department of Mental Hygiene, Charles W. Pilgrim. On October 1, 1931, Pilgrim State Hospital officially opened its doors as a facility. Dr. George Smith, superintendent of Central Islip, was appointed the acting superintendent of Pilgrim and conducted opening exercises. On November 5, 1931, the first 100 patients arrived at Building 1 from Central Islip. Dr. William J. Tiffany was appointed superintendent of the hospital on November 16, 1931, concurrently serving in the same capacity at Kings Park State Hospital. By June 30, 1932, about 1,970 patients were residing at Pilgrim State, having been transferred from other state hospitals.

Pilgrim State grew beyond its intended capacity, eventually housing 14,874 patients in the mid-1950s, making it the largest mental hospital in recorded history. Simultaneously, an additional 18,000 patients resided at the nearby Central Islip and Kings Park State Hospitals. With less than 11 miles separating each, these three facilities put Long Island on the map in the 1950s as a center of mental health care in the United States and the world. The year 1955 brought the drug chlorpromazine, marketed under the brand name Thorazine, which introduced neuroleptic drugs to the country. This and other pharmacological-based treatments led many professionals to believe mental illness could be managed more effectively. So effectively, in fact, that it was assumed antipsychotics would act as insulin does to a diabetic. Within the first few years of prescribing psychiatric medication as standard practice, it was clear that the symptoms for many individuals were ameliorated. Thousands of others, however, remained resistant to medication-based treatment. For a variety of reasons both good and bad, Pres. John F. Kennedy signed into law the Community Mental Health Act in 1963, creating a policy of deinstitutionalization nationwide. As drug therapy took hold of the frontline of psychiatric treatment, moral and activity-based therapies became increasingly scarce in the 1970s. Later that decade, all the state hospitals were renamed psychiatric centers, and the state hospital farms were no longer operational due to federal regulations prohibiting unpaid work by patients. The facilities became increasingly more stagnant, oriented more toward programs held indoors on locked wards as the population steadily decreased year after year.

A new paradigm known as the psychiatric rehabilitation model came to New York's psychiatric centers in the late 1970s, beginning at Willard Psychiatric Center with piece work. Programs aimed at social reintegration, vocational training, and symptom management were key tenets of this model, which replaced the medical model of care that began in the 1940s. In fall of 1996, after over a century of caring for mentally ill patients, Central Islip and Kings Park Psychiatric Center were shuttered, consolidating into Pilgrim Psychiatric Center. Although public mental health continues to evolve, the legacy of care and devotion to patients continues through present programs chartered at the former institutions.

One

From Farm Colonies to Hospitals

It is doubtful the founding staff of Kings Park and Central Islip could have imagined that the two facilities would grow to house over 18,000 patients combined in dozens of brick buildings at their peak. In the first months, when 55 men and women arrived at the St. Johnland Farm colony consisting of a temporary wooden building and an old barn for living quarters, Supt. John C. Shore remarked, "The arrangements there are of the most primitive kind, and it is very unsatisfactory caring for them in this manner. At first many of the patients ran away . . . and I am at present obligated to have one of my assistant physicians constantly there."

In its infancy at Central Islip, the New York City Farm Colony for the Insane faced similar challenges. However, with the labor of both staff and patients in the pioneer days, both colonies grew from an abject wilderness into well-established facilities. In 1891, the railroad changed the station name at St. Johnland to Kings Park, which the town took its name from. On September 22, 1898, Kings Park graduated its first class of nurses from the facility, with an additional 14 graduating from a similar program at Central Islip that year. The institutions attracted many Irish immigrants, especially in Kings Park, who worked there and settled in adjoining towns. By the early 1900s, each state hospital had independent medical surgical accommodations, various shops, powerhouses, a full-scale farm, ward buildings, and many other ancillary buildings. The institutions were largely self-sustaining, producing as much as two-thirds of the food consumed there as well as sundries such as clothing and shoes.

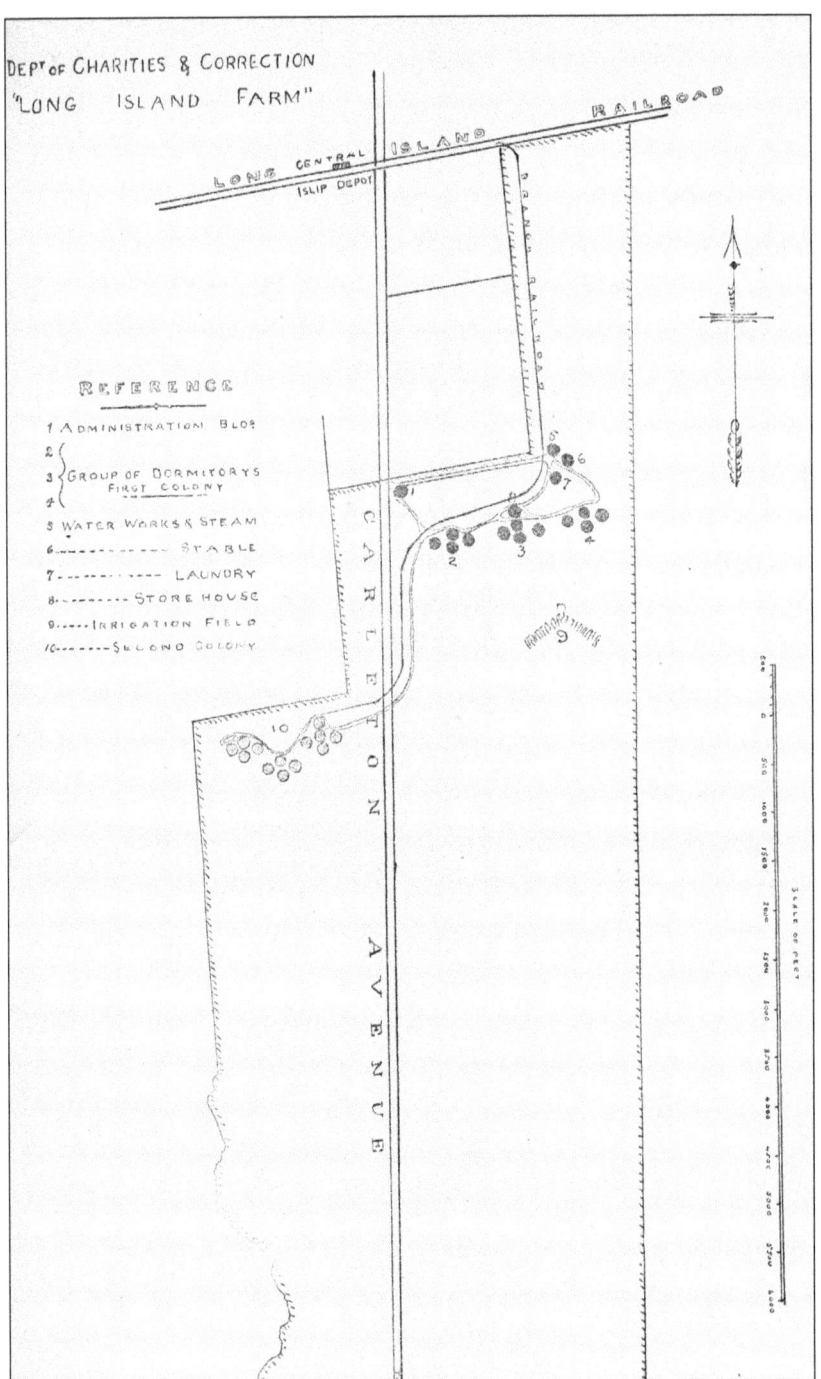

This is an 1887 hand-drawn map for the new colony at Central Islip during the period of administration by the New York City Board of Charities and Correction. The dark circles represent the buildings to be constructed first, followed by those indicated by light circles. As previously mentioned, the rationale was to rely on the mother asylums on Hart and Blackwell Islands for as many services (such as laundry) as could be allowed until the success of the colony was evaluated. These groups would make up the initial "farm colony" at Central Islip.

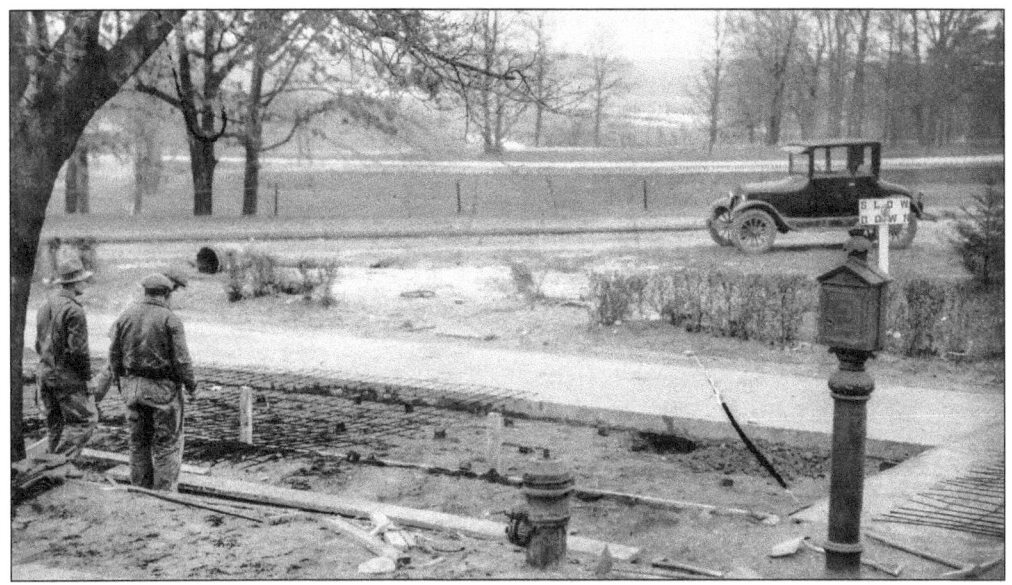

Initially, farm colony roads were unpaved, long and windy stretches. When it rained, wheels would often get stuck in muddy ruts. By the late 1920s, most of the main roads at Kings Park were surfaced with concrete and bluestone curbs. Above, men lay a new concrete roadway over "the Boulevard" in 1925, the well-known main stretch of road through the hospital campus still used by locals today. Below, men are moving wet concrete using wheelbarrows. Even for tradesmen performing manual labor, appearance was critical, and modest dress was enforced on the grounds.

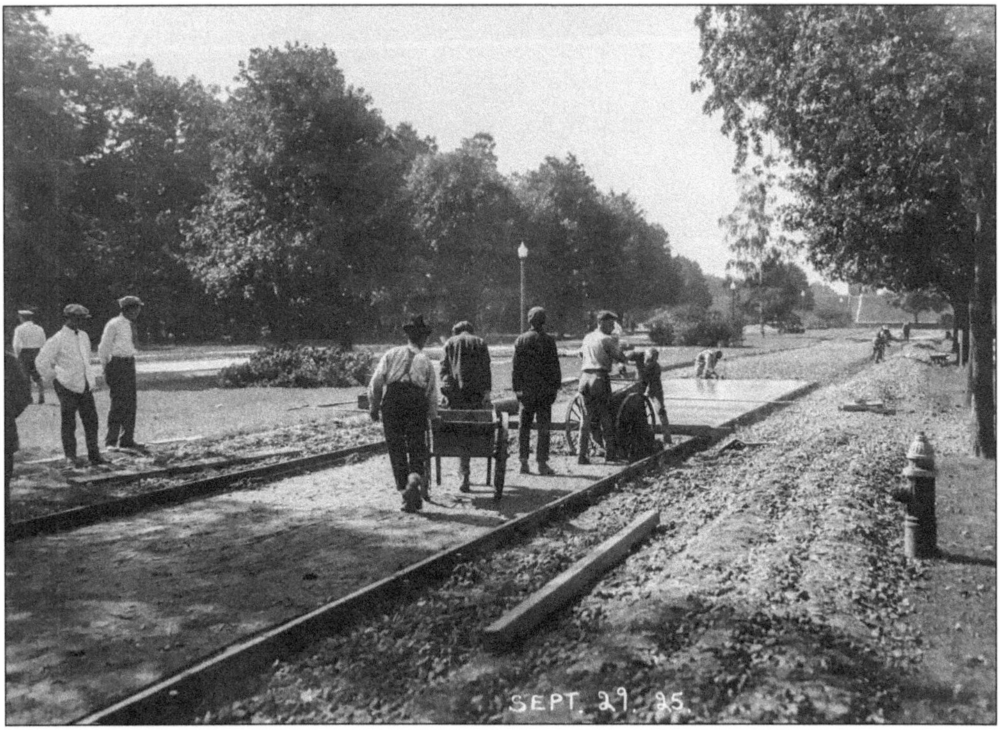

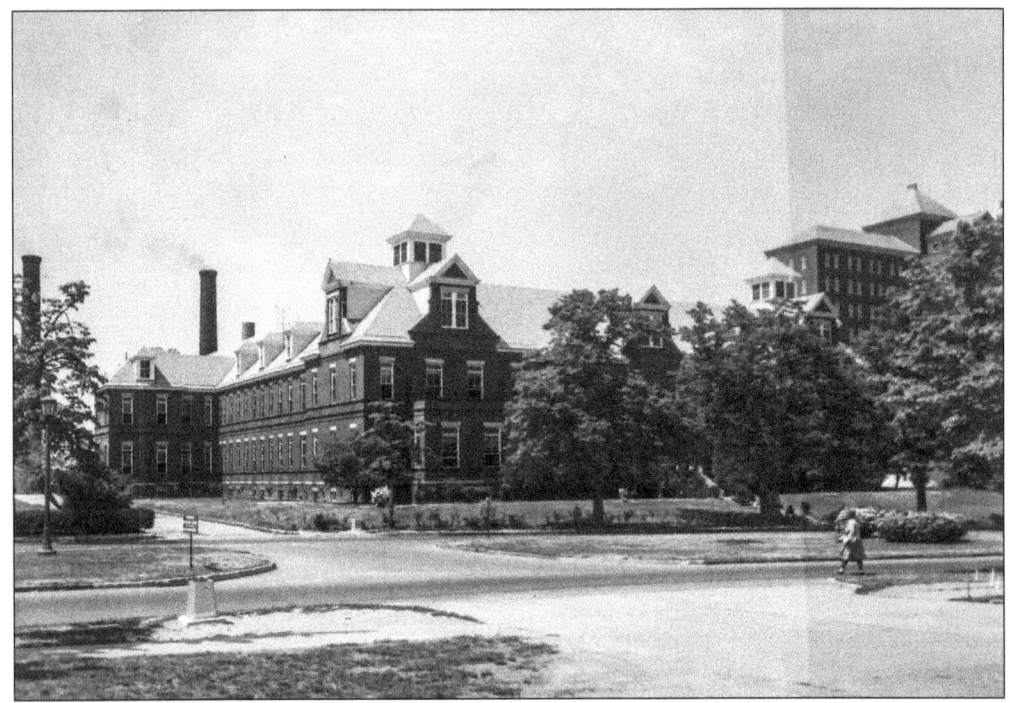

In this 1965 view facing north, Building 11, or "Building C," on Kings Park Boulevard is at center. Slightly to the north in the background, the monumental Building 93, a geriatric infirmary at the time, is visible. To the west, the twin smokestacks of the second powerhouse can be seen.

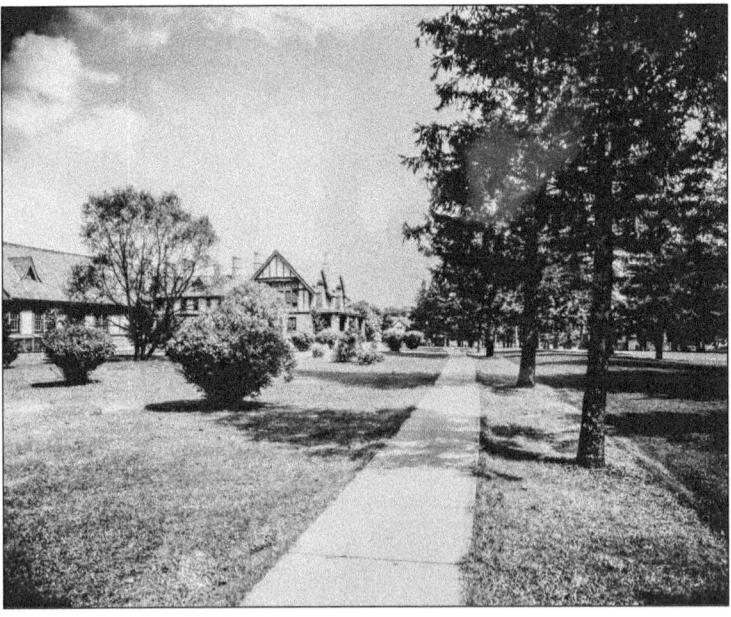

Construction seemed to be without end at Central Islip for many decades after its inception. Although the style of buildings varied from decade to decade, as well as the population each unit was planned for, ornate details and tranquil grounds always remained at the front of the planners' minds. Here, one of the ward buildings in the Smith Group is pictured in the 1920s.

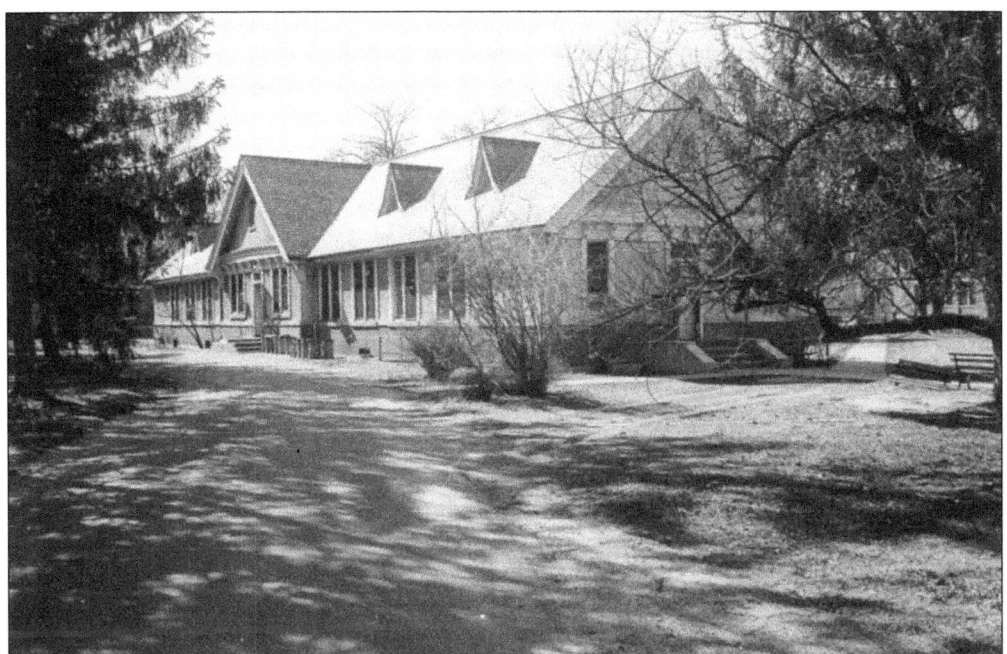

Just to the north of the Smith Group was the MacGregor Group of wards. Like its sister cluster across the grassy quad, it consisted of three main wards and a central dining hall. Shown here is Building 37D, the dining hall for the group. This building remains today as a recreation center for the apartment units constructed over the old grounds of Central Islip State Hospital.

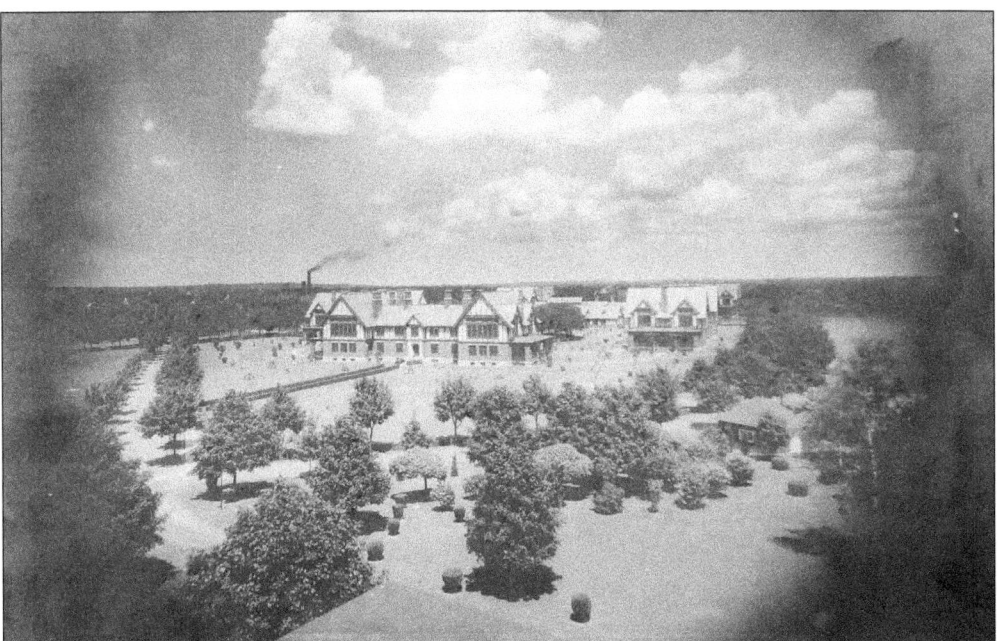

Looking southwest across the colony grounds, the Smith Group is in full view. In the distance, coal smoke from the powerhouse is visible. Patients spent much time outdoors here, engaging in physical and social activity on the well-manicured, park-like grounds. The Smith Group was named for Dr. George Smith, a revered superintendent of the colony.

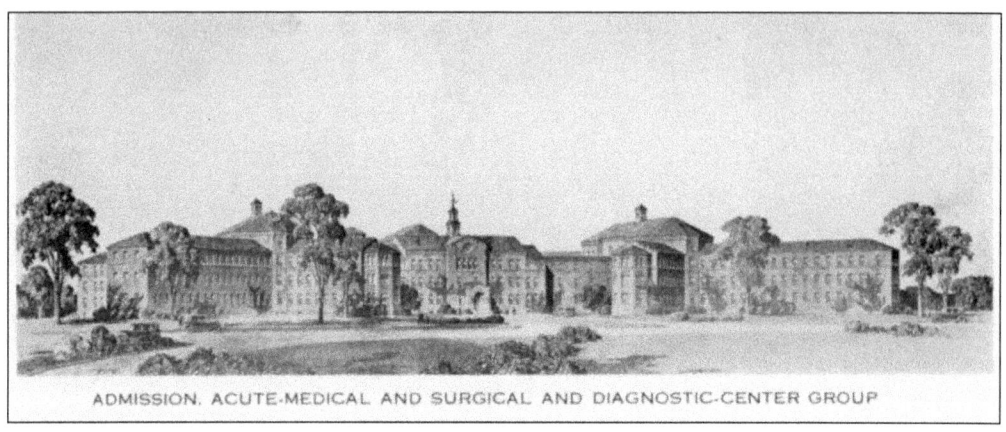

ADMISSION, ACUTE-MEDICAL AND SURGICAL AND DIAGNOSTIC-CENTER GROUP

Pilgrim State Hospital was devised during a time when the legislature was in tune with the need to supply secure but salubrious settings for the mentally ill of New York. The Long Island facilities housed and treated patients from all five boroughs of New York City, as well as both counties of Long Island until 1974. By then, Pilgrim State was primarily admitting patients from Nassau County. Shown above is the architect's pencil drawing of Building 23 (center), Pilgrim's state-of-the-art medical hospital, school of nursing, and surgical unit. Flanking it were Buildings 22 and 24, used for male and female admissions. Below is a rendering of one cluster consisting of four ward buildings with a central kitchen, all connected by an underground passage and arranged in a quad.

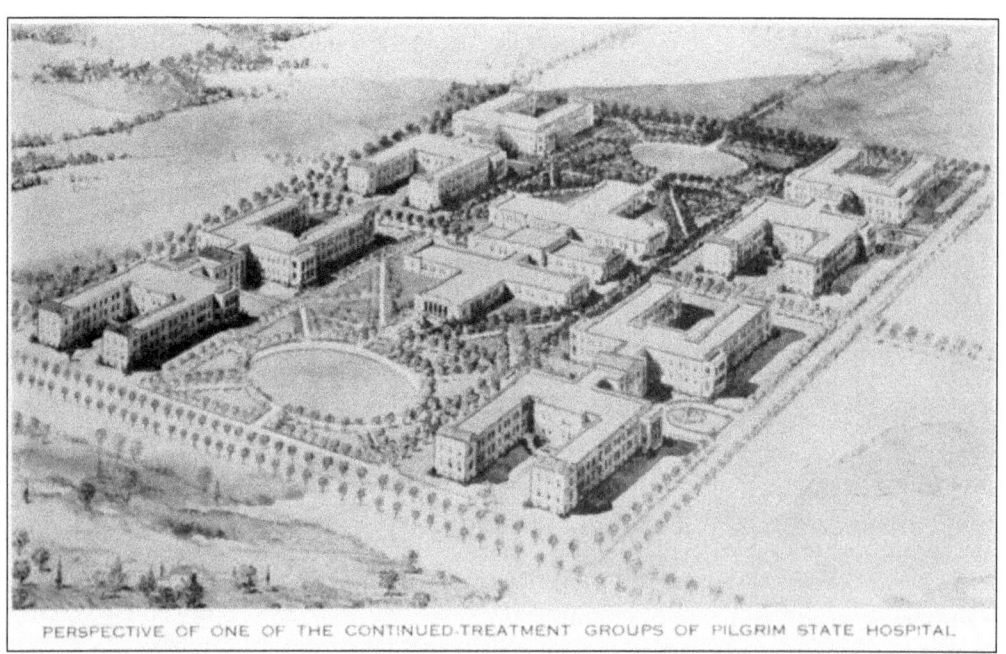

PERSPECTIVE OF ONE OF THE CONTINUED-TREATMENT GROUPS OF PILGRIM STATE HOSPITAL

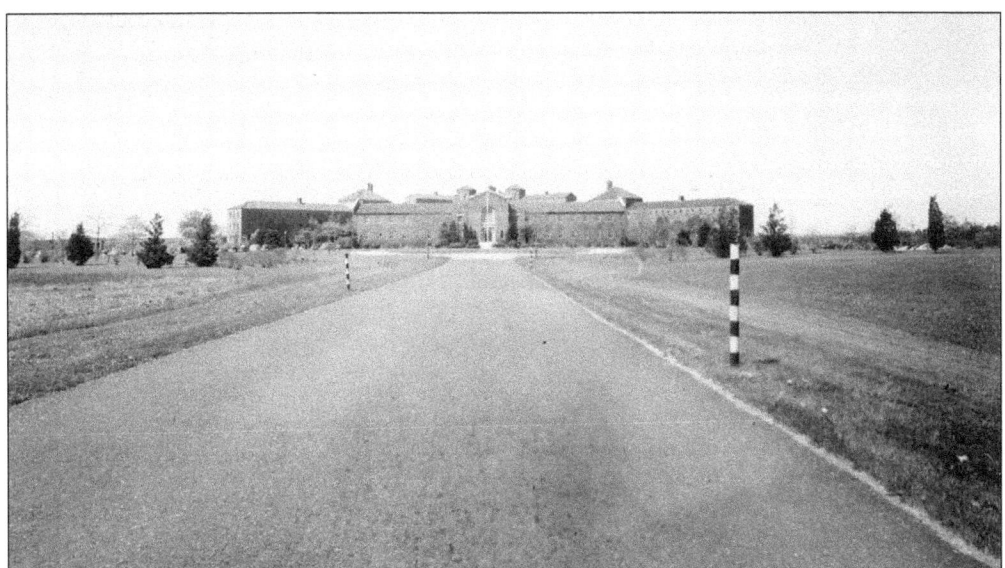

Upon entering the grounds of Pilgrim State off the Sagtikos Parkway, Building 18 was the first structure to catch the eye. Building 18 was Pilgrim's administration unit. Here, the director of the hospital, as well as other personnel of rank, had offices until 2001, when the building was closed and sold off along with a large parcel of hospital land.

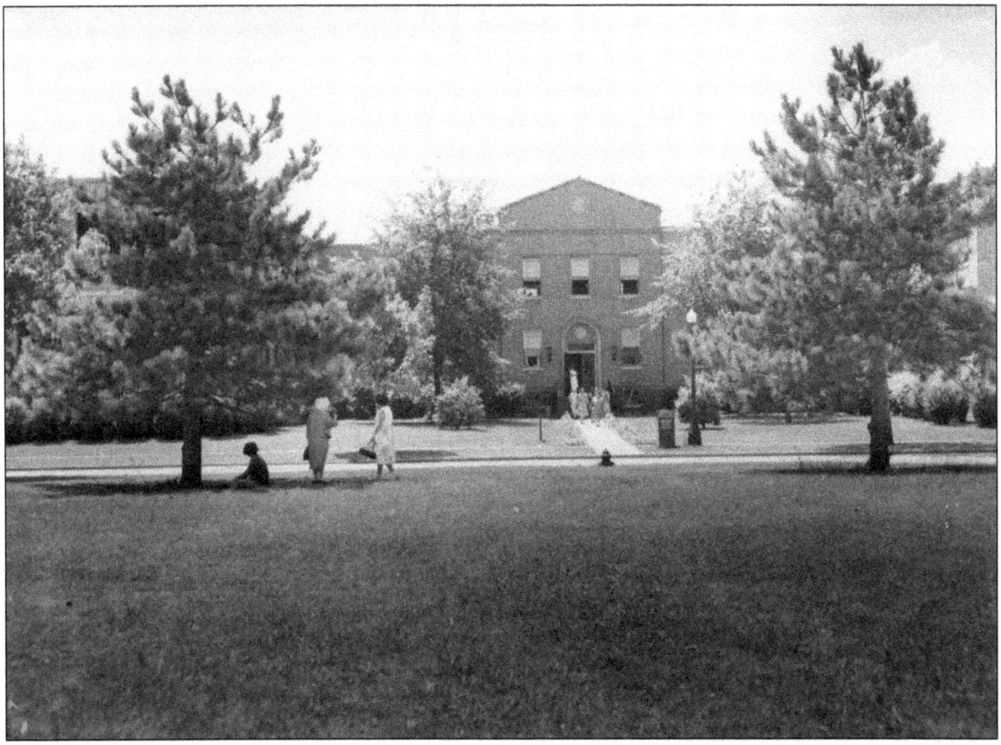

The two-story ward buildings at Pilgrim were sometimes referred to as "H Dorms" by some senior staff due to their H-shaped appearance from overhead. In the opening days of the hospital through the 1970s, each side of the campus was separated by sex. The women seen here are outside Building 6, part of the female cluster of wards on the campus.

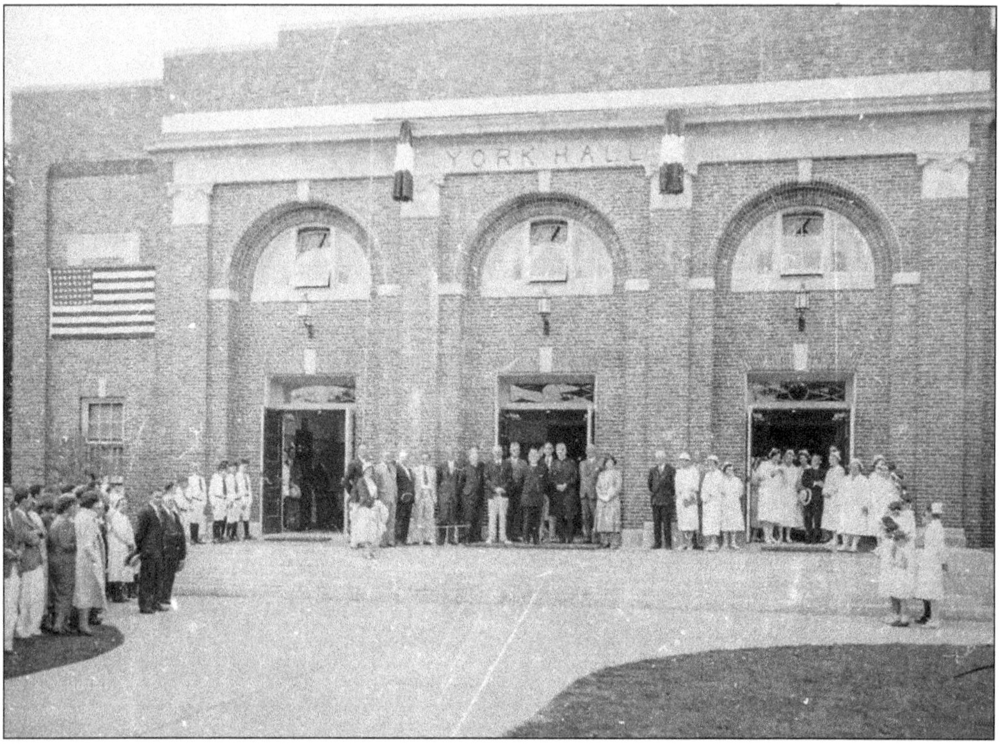

York Hall at Kings Park was built for recreation activity. Both patients and staff enjoyed attending its many social, sports, and holiday functions. Movie projectors for playing films were located on the second-floor balcony. Accommodations for a full court basketball game, as well as a stage, were located inside. Holiday meals were held at York Hall in addition to nursing school graduation exercises and religious services.

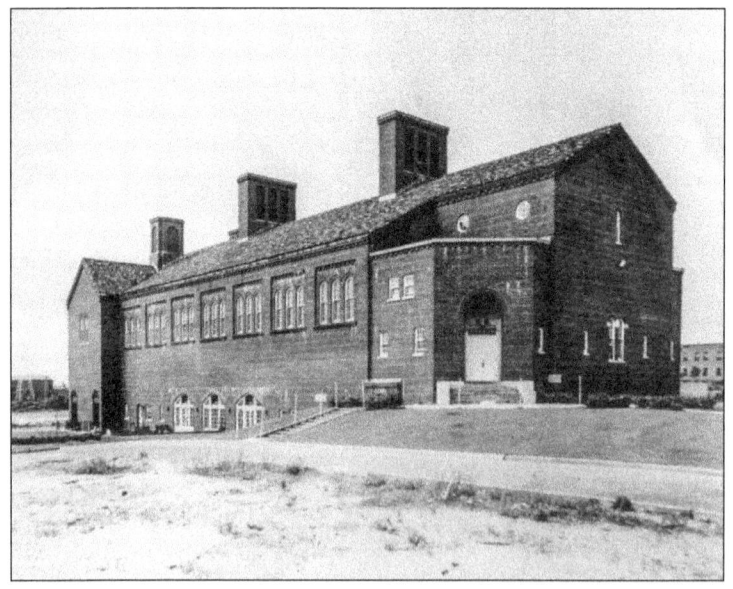

The assembly hall building at Pilgrim State was similar architecturally to the other hospitals. Inside was a community store on the lower level, a stage on the first floor, full basketball court, and balcony seating. The assembly hall was the only place patients and staff were permitted to fraternize with members of the opposite sex during the days of gender segregation at the hospital.

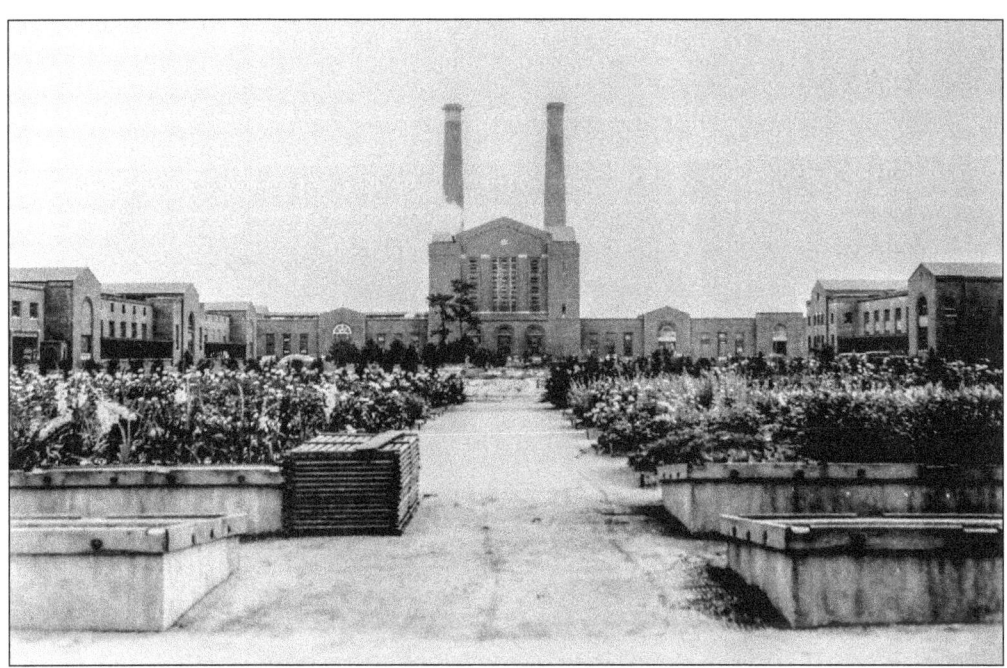

From the beginning, each facility generated its own steam and electricity. In the early days, power plants were coal-fired until the advent of commercial oil and gas fuels. Coal came by barge early on at Kings Park until the railroad was routed directly onto the hospital campus. At Central Islip, Pilgrim, and Edgewood, coal came by rail from day one. Building 35, Pilgrim's power plant, can be seen in the distance above. Flowers in the foreground were being grown in beds by patients and staff for use on the grounds. Below is the power plant for Edgewood State Hospital, a division of Pilgrim State just a mile up the road.

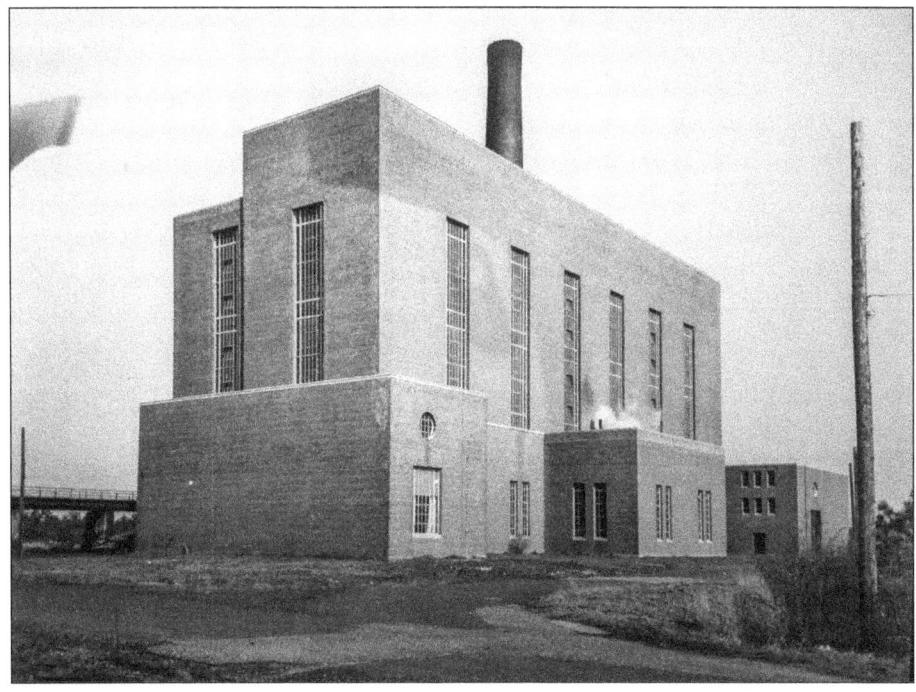

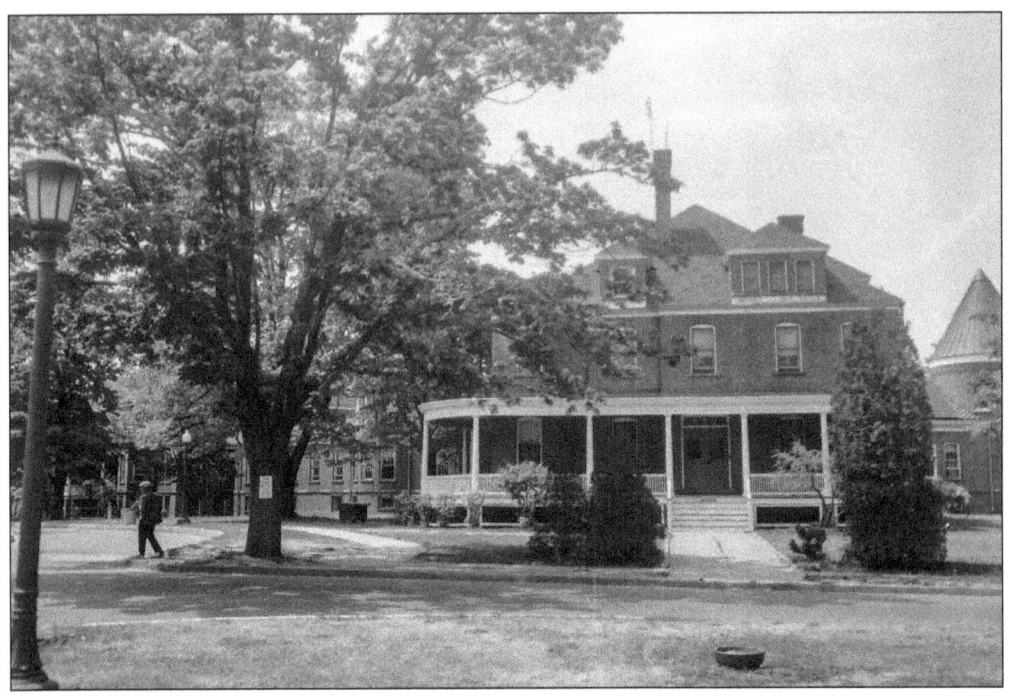

While Kings Park was under the jurisdiction of Kings County Asylum in Brooklyn, the administration had to communicate between both facilities through mail carried by horse until the advent of the telegraph. This was the administration building at Kings Park State Hospital, located in the front of Group I, pictured in the 1910s. When it became commercially available, a telegraph was installed here to communicate with the Brooklyn asylum.

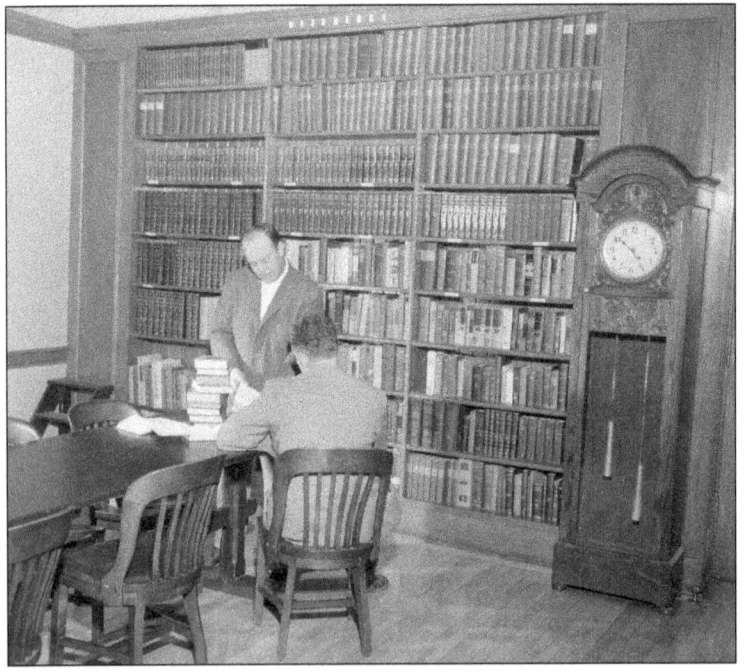

Libraries were a resource of great importance at the hospitals, especially during the days of geographical isolation. Reference copies of journals, encyclopedias, and the material needed for those attending nursing school at the institutions could be found here. This 1950s photograph shows the staff library in Robbins Hall at Central Islip.

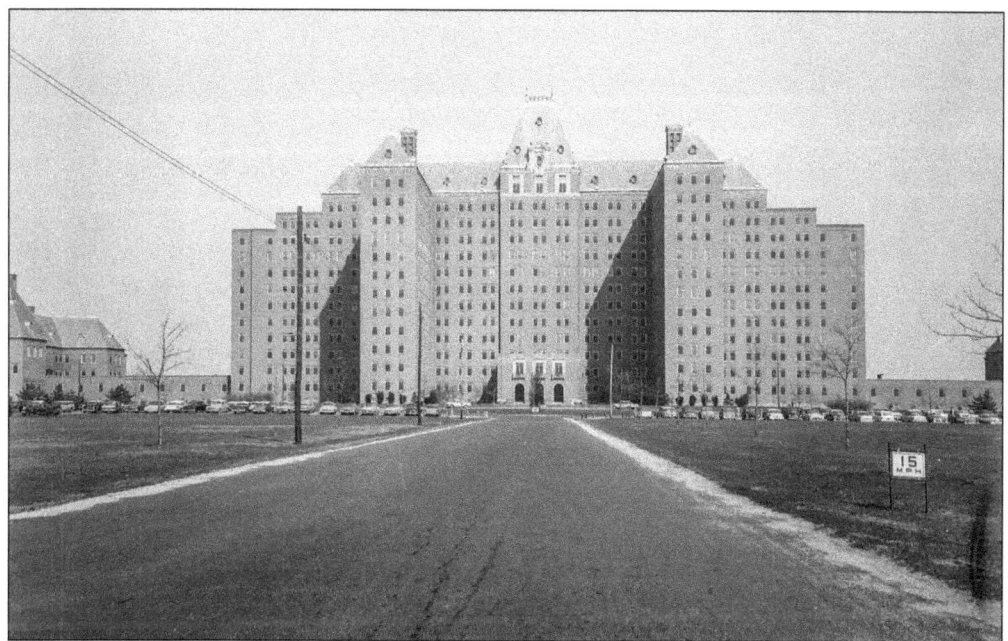

Pilgrim and Edgewood were the only two Long Island facilities to open with large, high-rise buildings for the care of patients. Shortly after opening, it was clear that the need for inpatient beds versus room on the ground was a problem; the solution was to build upward. Building 102 at Edgewood (above) was the tallest ward building constructed for the Long Island state hospitals. It contained all of the admission services, recreation, medical, diagnostic, and x-ray units necessary to run the facility. Although never built to full scale, Edgewood was utilized as a tuberculosis center for mentally ill patients from other state institutions all over New York after World War II until the 1960s. Building 25, shown below at Pilgrim State, opened as a continuing treatment building with the rest of the campus.

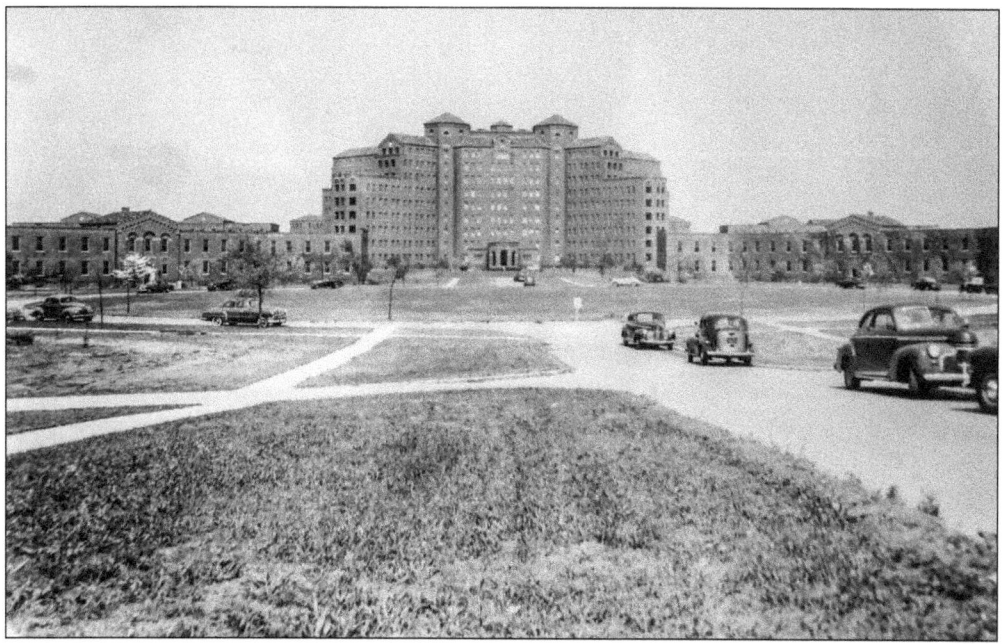

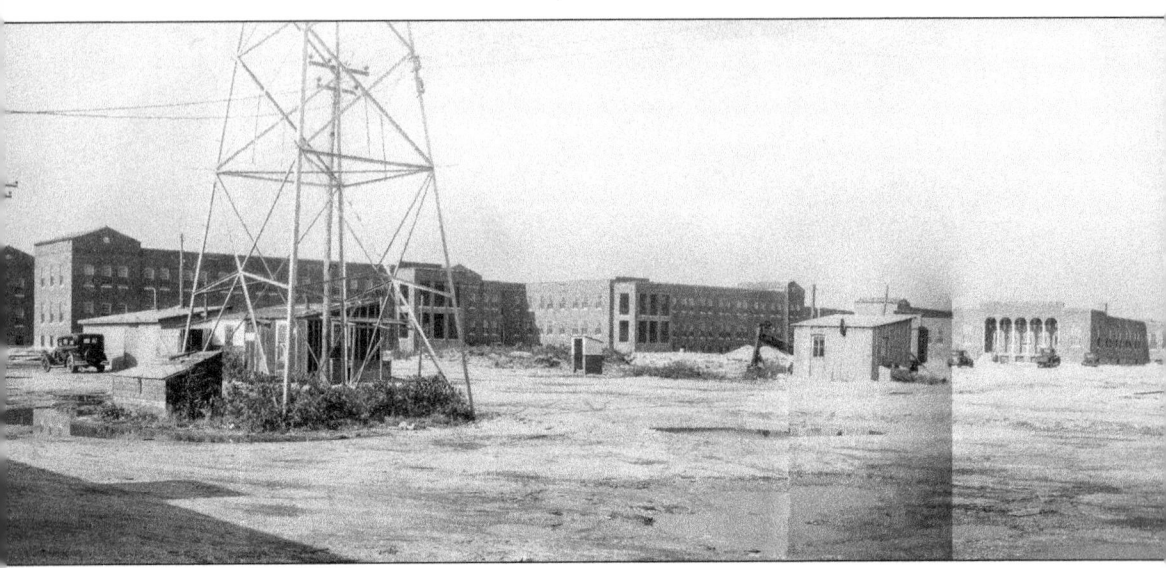

Construction on Pilgrim State was different from Kings Park and Central Islip, in that for the most part, the buildings were planned and constructed at the same time. This allowed for a grid of roadways on the grounds and proportional spacing between buildings. Kings Park and Central Islip were built sporadically, meaning available lots of land between previously existing structures

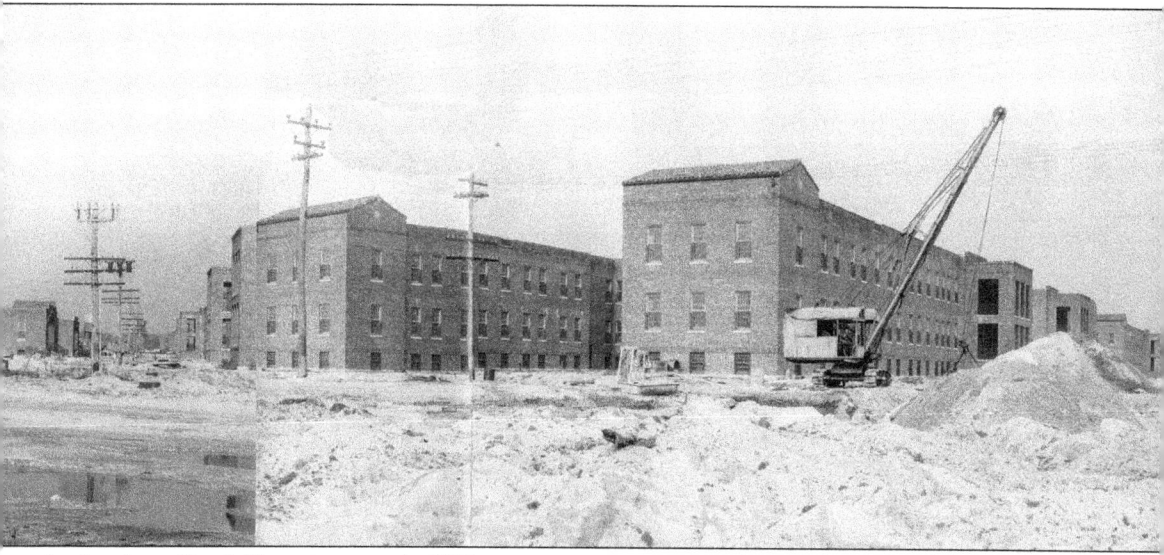

had to be utilized. Here, in an early 1930s construction image, a cluster of wards with a central kitchen is shown. The roads on the grounds were not yet paved in concrete, but are distinguishable. Also visible are overhead power lines, which, upon completion of the facility, were buried in underground conduits, allowing for unobstructed views on the grounds.

In this 1950s image, a white building well known by a generation of staff now long passed at Kings Park State Hospital stands in the foreground. This building was used for employee recreation after being decommissioned as a cottage for patients' quarters. In the background towers Building 93. The "white house" cottage was demolished sometime in the 1970s, along with other wooden structures lining the boulevard.

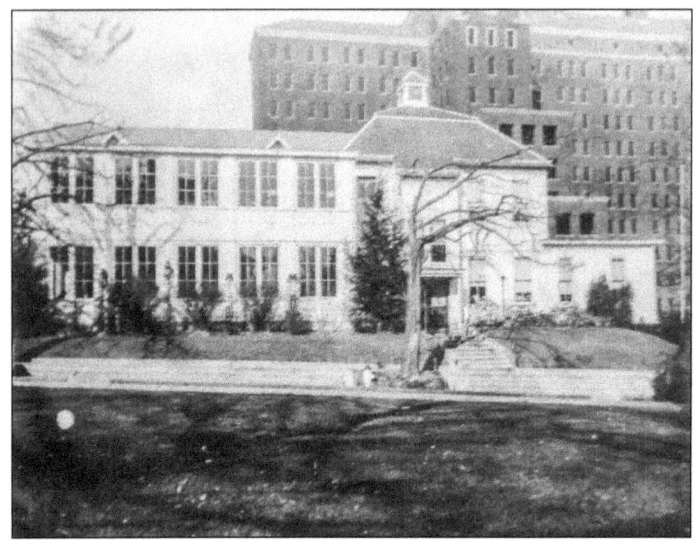

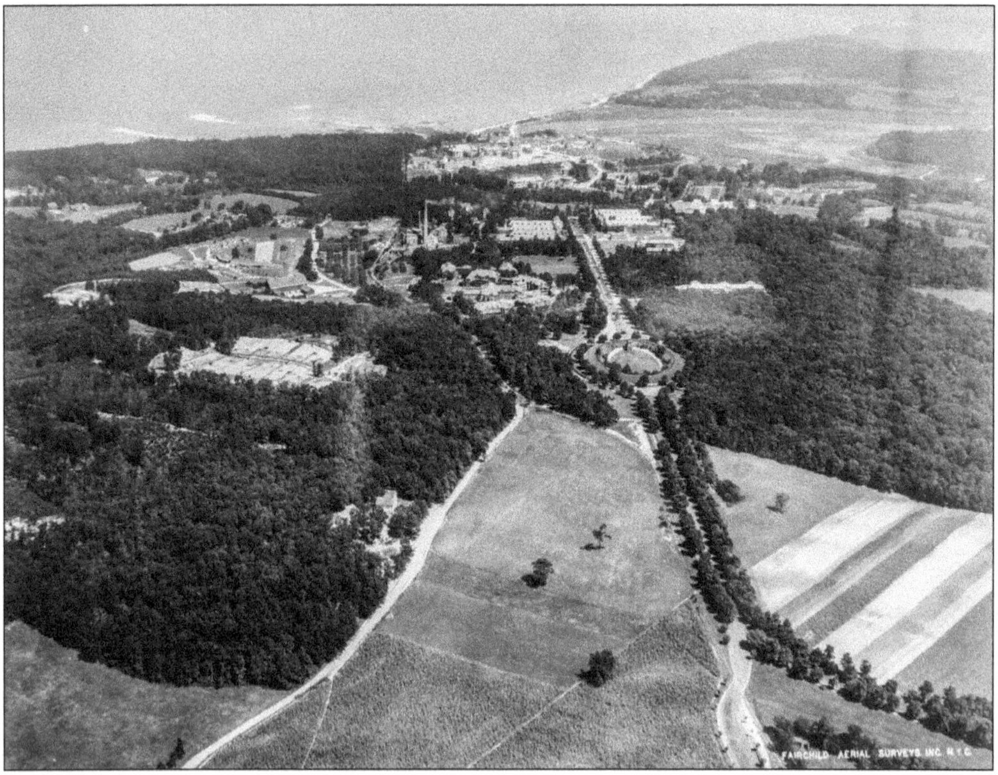

This aerial view of Kings Park shows the grounds before the construction of buildings taller than four stories. At center, a circular area can be seen on the main stretch of road. This was an early water reservoir on the grounds that supplied gravity-fed water to the first buildings. With the advent of taller structures, it was removed, and a tall water tower was added.

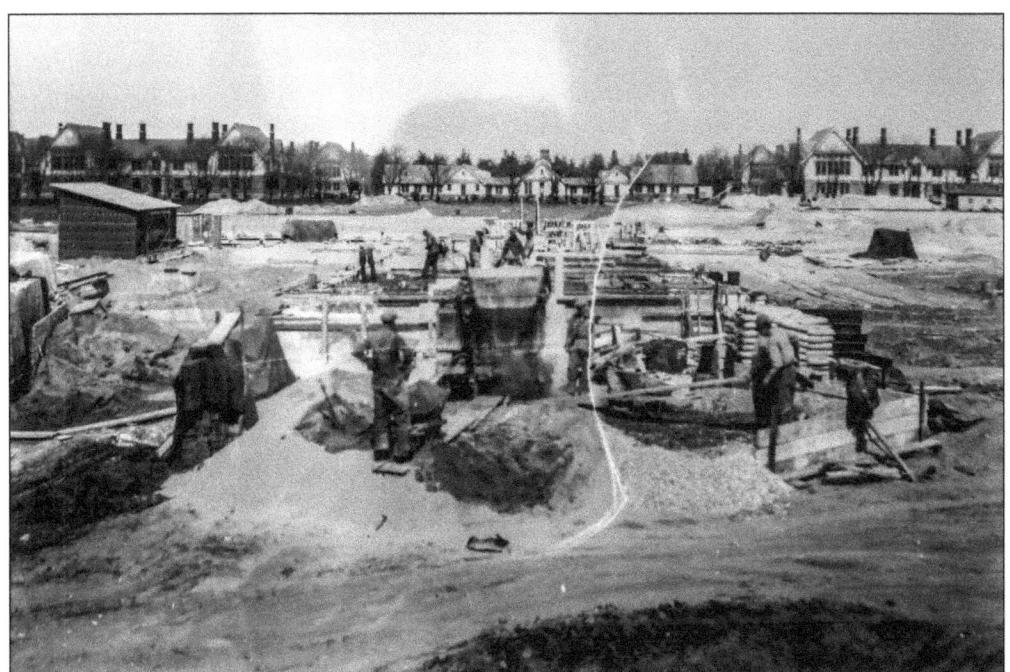

Construction projects at Central Islip continued into the 1980s with the addition of buildings for outpatient use as the hospital census dwindled. In the earlier part of the 20th century, however, growth was staggering. Here, in an early image, men can be seen working on the foundation of the final building to be constructed in the MacGregor group of wards.

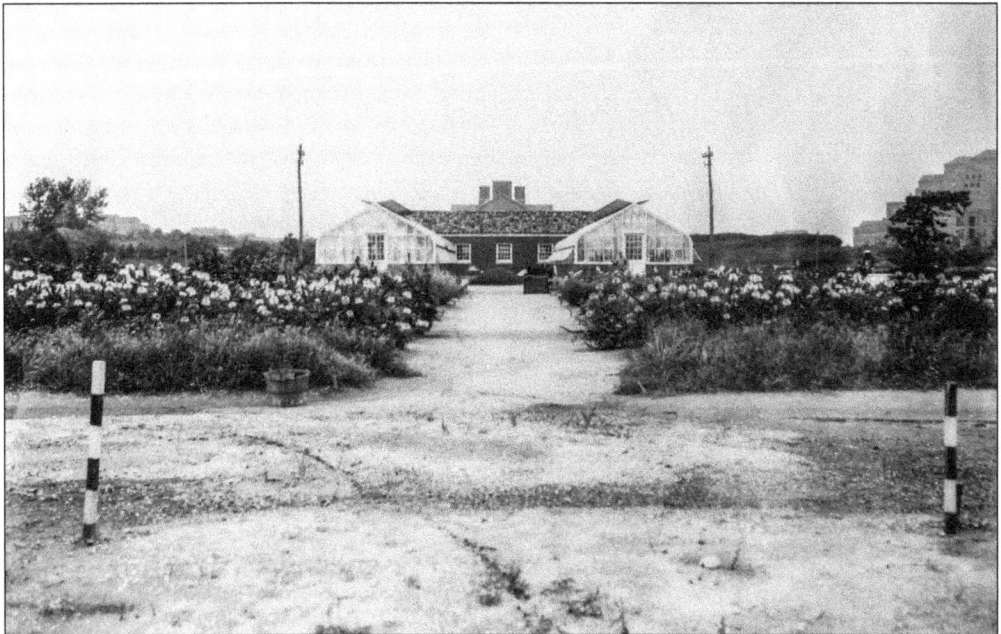

The hospital greenhouses were a source of pride for the facility and provided therapeutic activity for patients. Little cost was involved in running these buildings. Since steam was being pumped all over the campuses for heating, running a steam line to these buildings involved minimal additional expense. This 1940s photograph shows the greenhouse at Pilgrim State in the spring.

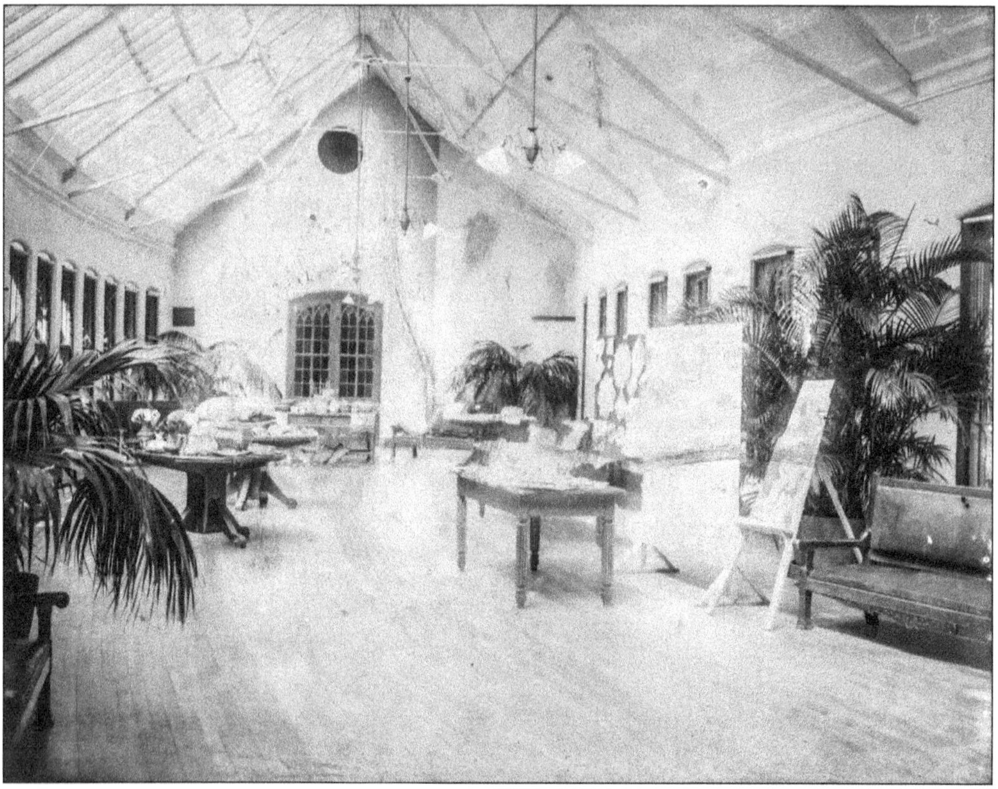

Group I at Kings Park was perhaps one of the hospital's most ornate buildings constructed in the 20th century. Connecting the different wards and administrative sections of the building were tall, glass-ceilinged breezeways that were lined with greenery all year long. They were in fact so large they doubled as areas for daily activity and social events. Visible in this 1910s image is a section of Group I's connecting corridors. (Courtesy of the Kings Park Heritage Museum.)

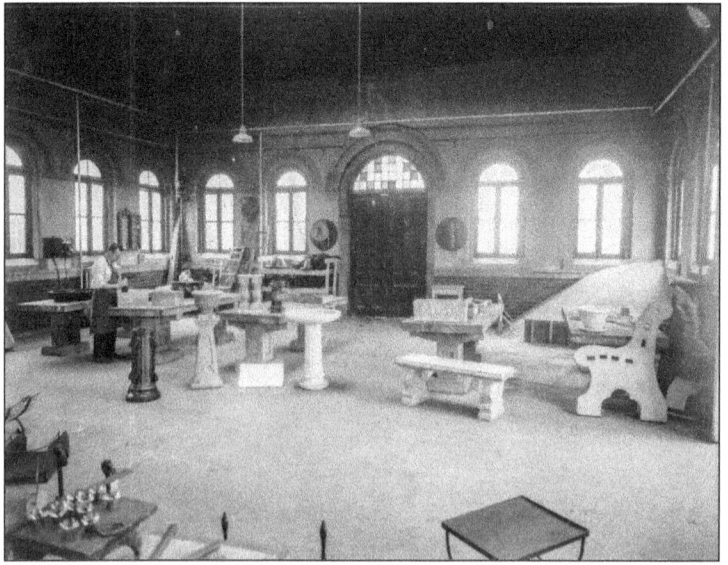

This small brick building at Kings Park State Hospital saw many uses over the years. Constructed in the 1890s as a shoe shop, the structure reminded under the administration of the activities department. In this 1925 image, a man can be seen working on masonry projects. The space was used to cast cement molds for everything from small benches to garden ornaments to bird baths.

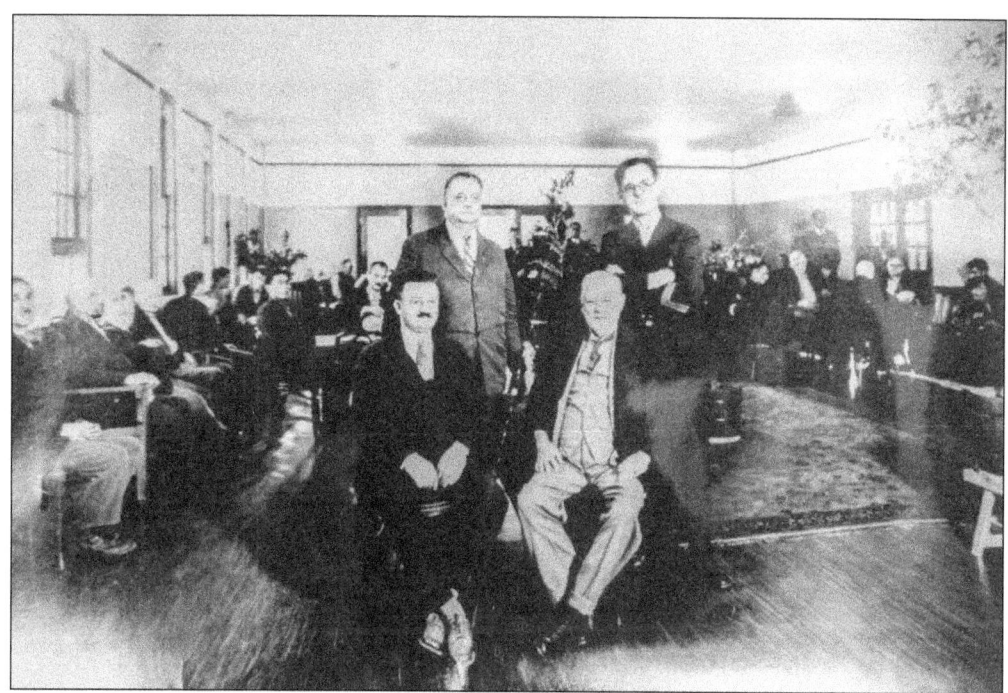

A ward at the Central Islip State Hospital is seen here in the early 1910s. Above are men of the hospital administration. In the first row at far right is Dr. George Smith. Dr. Smith was a legend at Central Islip. Beginning his career as a superintendent at Central Islip in the days of the City Farm colony, Smith stayed on staff until 1932. He was even appointed first superintendent when Pilgrim State Hospital was commissioned, later replaced by Dr. Tiffany due to Smith's impending retirement after 50 years of service. Smith is credited with the development of Central Islip from an experimental colony into a successful and humane state hospital. He wrote many books on the benefits of recreation and vocational rehabilitation at Central Islip and was an exemplar of compassionate, individual-based treatment.

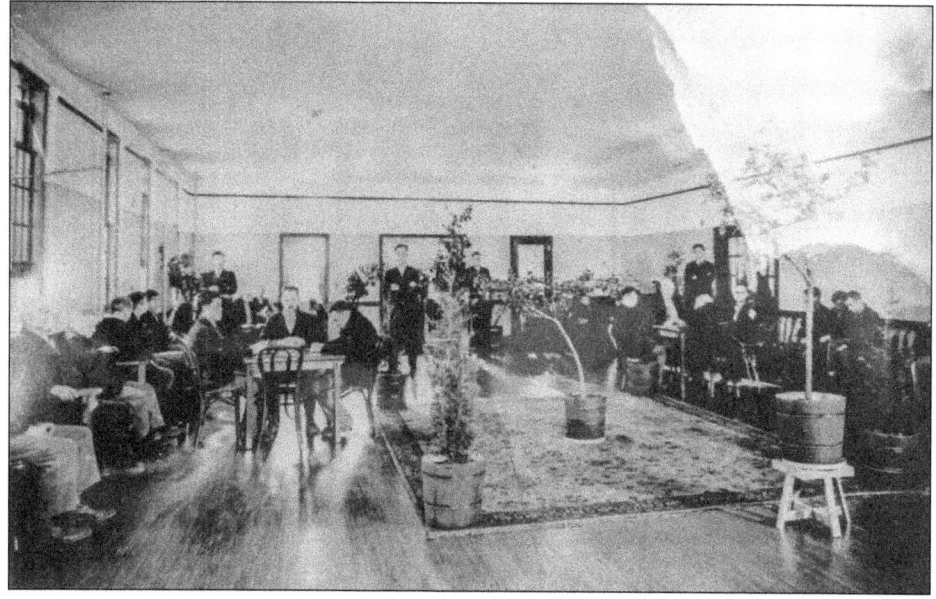

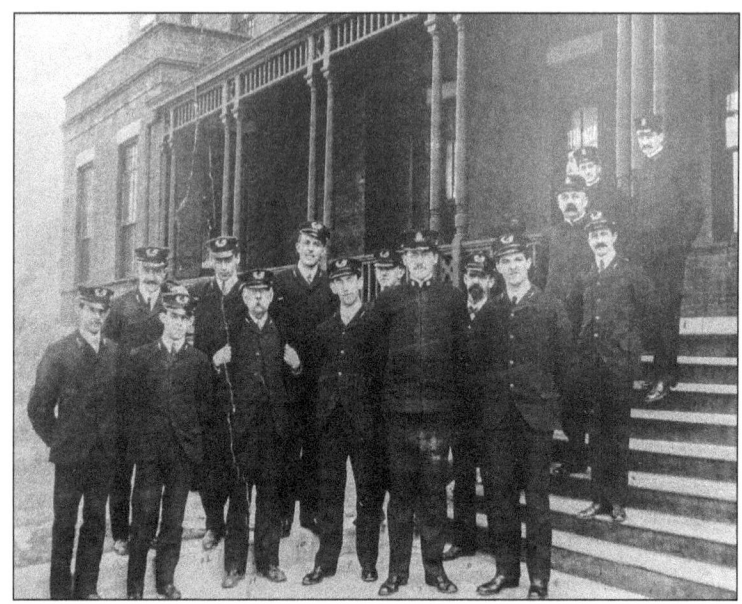

Pictured outside the front porch of the administration building in 1894 are the men who supervised Kings Park State Hospital. At the time, the rank of each member was worn on their collar. Administrators were referred to as officers of the hospital, as they held public office. Note the ornate detail work on the porch.

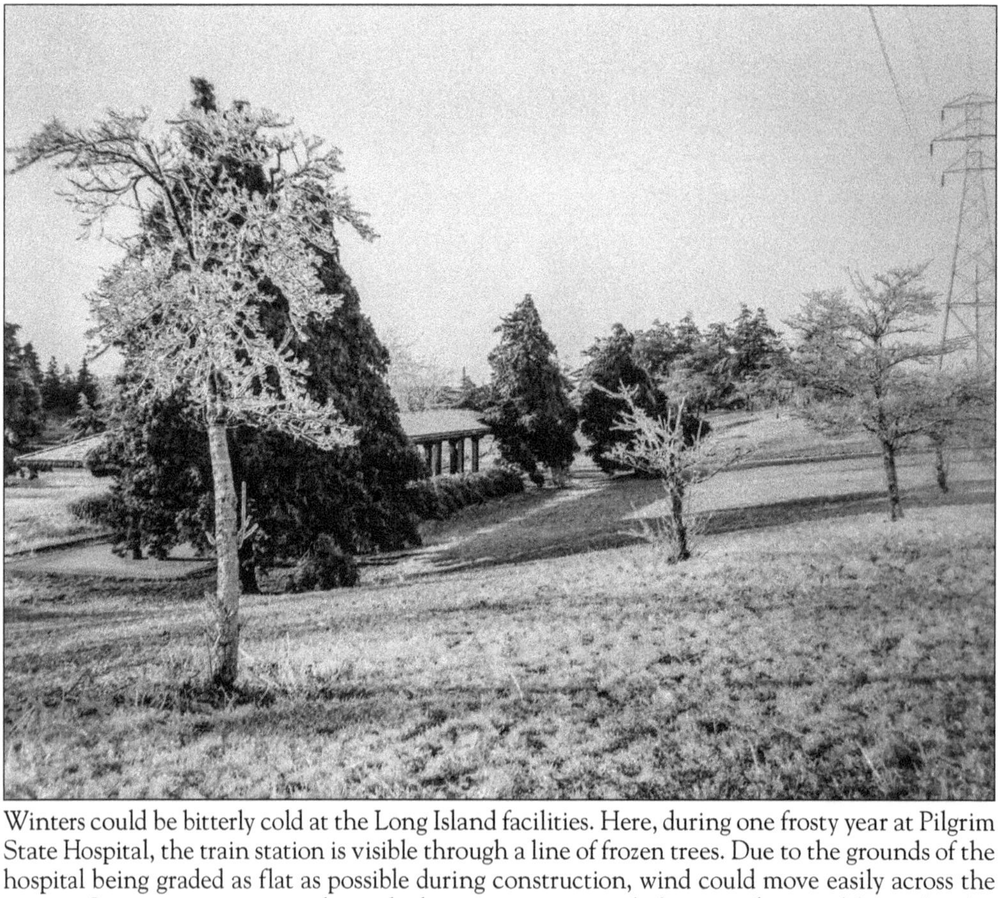

Winters could be bitterly cold at the Long Island facilities. Here, during one frosty year at Pilgrim State Hospital, the train station is visible through a line of frozen trees. Due to the grounds of the hospital being graded as flat as possible during construction, wind could move easily across the campus. It was not uncommon during bad storms to see snow drifts on roads several feet in height.

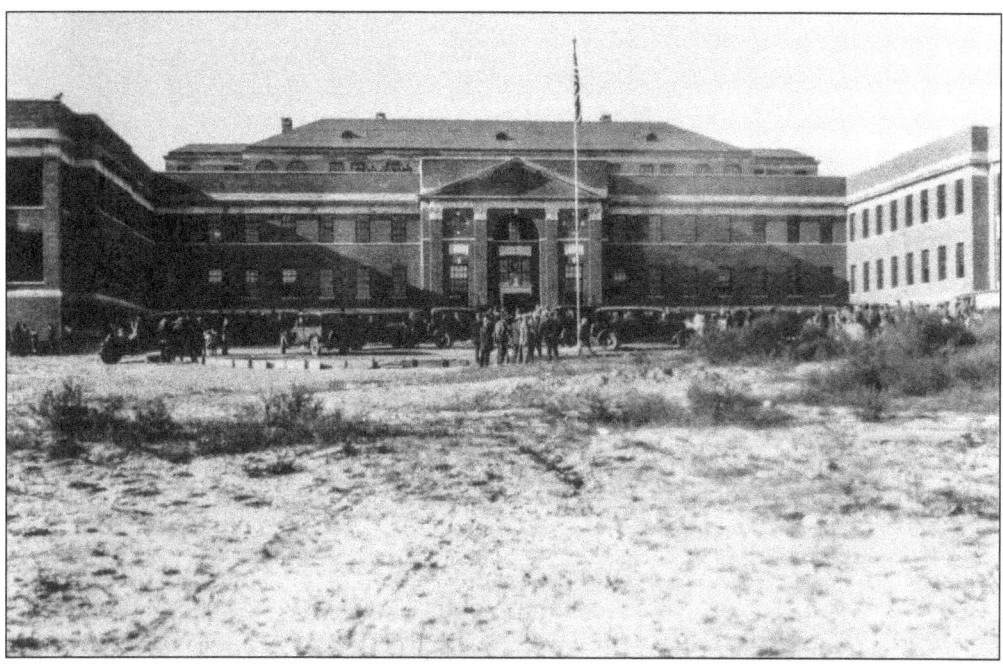

The Veterans Memorial Hospital at Kings Park was a group of 17 buildings constructed after World War I to treat soldiers who returned with mental impairments. The plan was that after the veterans were eventually returned to society, the buildings would stay in use as a memorial to their service and sacrifice. Sadly, World War II ensued shortly after, keeping these buildings open with their original purpose of treating servicemen. The photograph above was taken the day Building 136 opened in 1927 after a cost of $1 million. The uniformed men were from the National Guard. Below, a 1923 image taken at the ground-breaking ceremony of the building group shows projects completed by military service members at Kings Park. (Both, courtesy of the Kings Park Heritage Museum.)

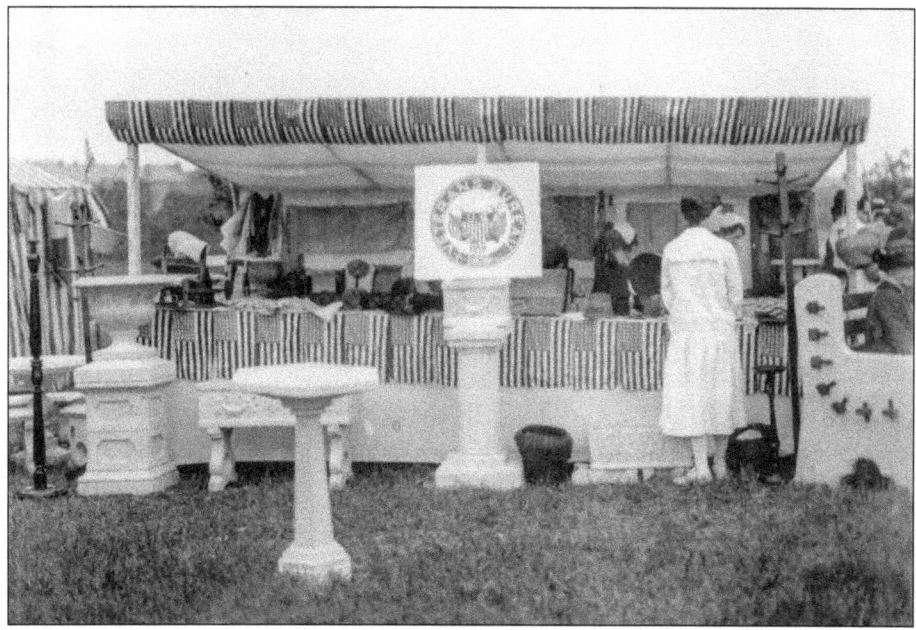

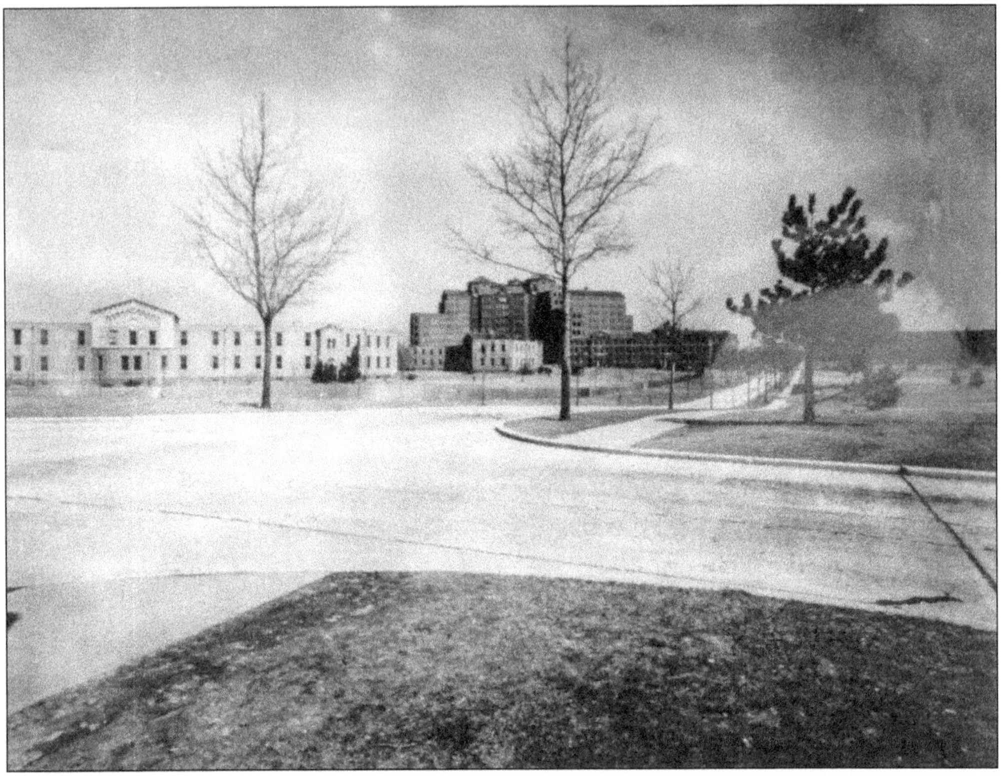

The grounds at Pilgrim State were built on a grid similar to New York City blocks. This 1960s image was taken at an intersection that still exists today. With the exception of vegetation growth, this view is largely unchanged today. In the distance, the tall Building 25 can be seen. It was built primarily to house older patients.

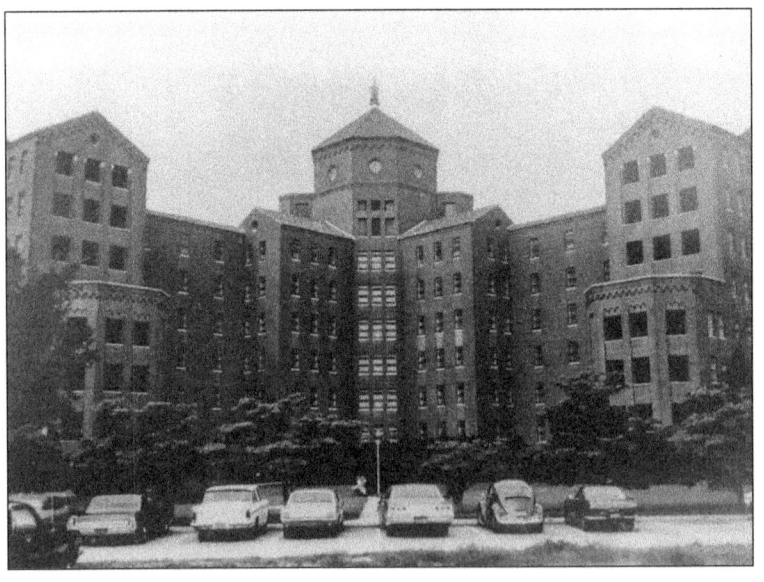

In this 1960s photograph, Pilgrim State's 80s group is seen with a row of vintage automobiles. The 80s group is currently the last building for the overnight lodging of state inpatients on the grounds of the hospital. At the time of this image, the porches at the ends of the wings allowed for fresh air on the ward.

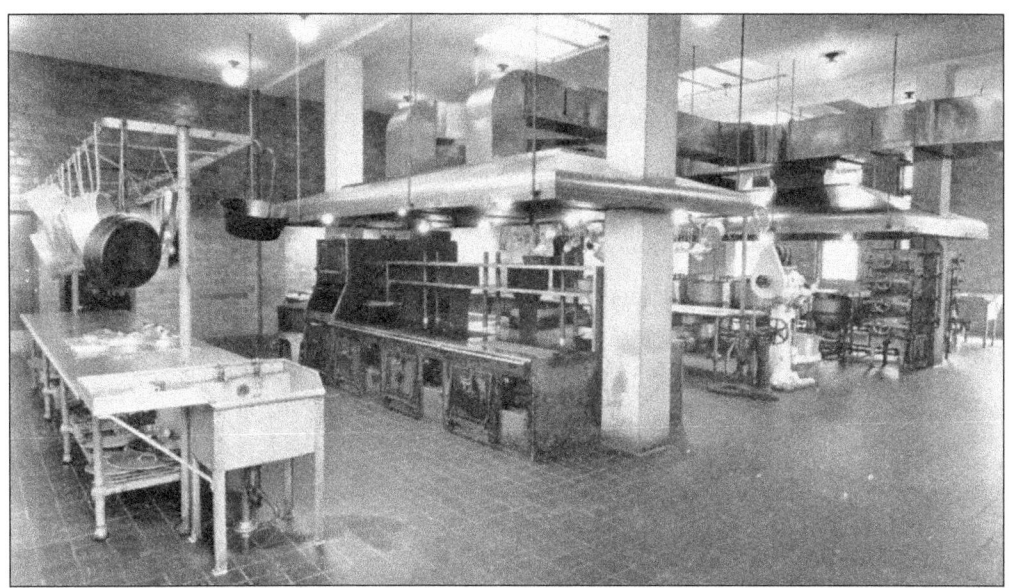

Food service at the institutions was a vital job that required long and laborious hours for modest pay. The hospital kitchens were responsible for preparing three meals and snacks daily for patients as well as employee meals in the earlier days. Independent bakeries on the grounds prepared bread and baked goods as well as specialty items on the holidays. When Pilgrim State Hospital was at its peak population of approximately 15,000 patients, the kitchens were required to serve three meals per day to all of them, plus staff. That is more than 45,000 meals daily, which was comparable to a small city. Above is one of the kitchens at Pilgrim. Below is a patient dining hall area.

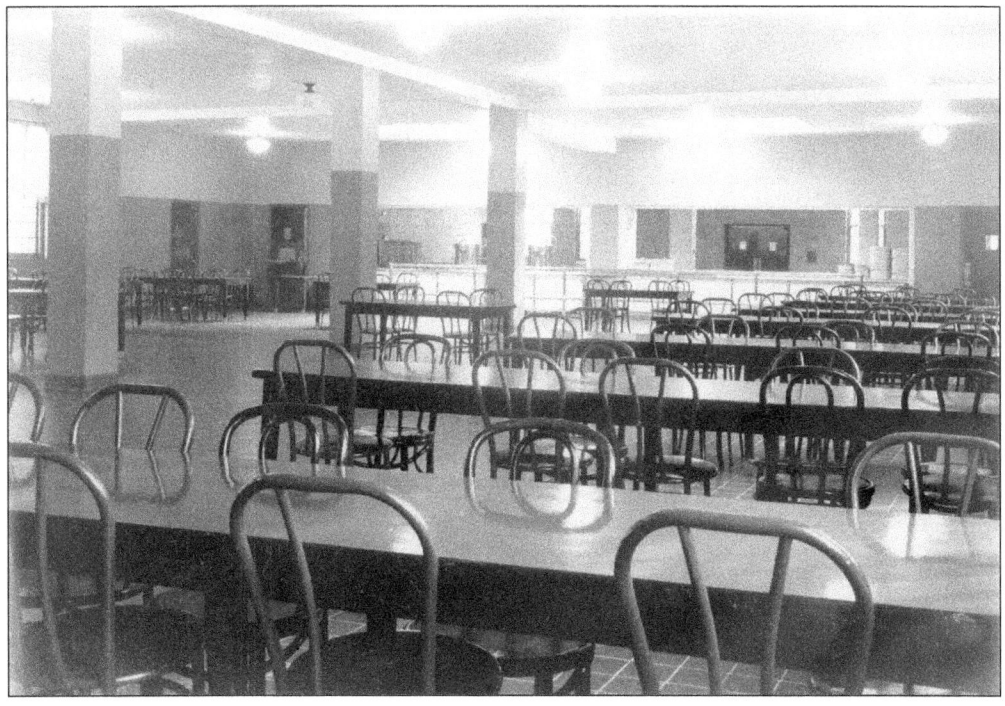

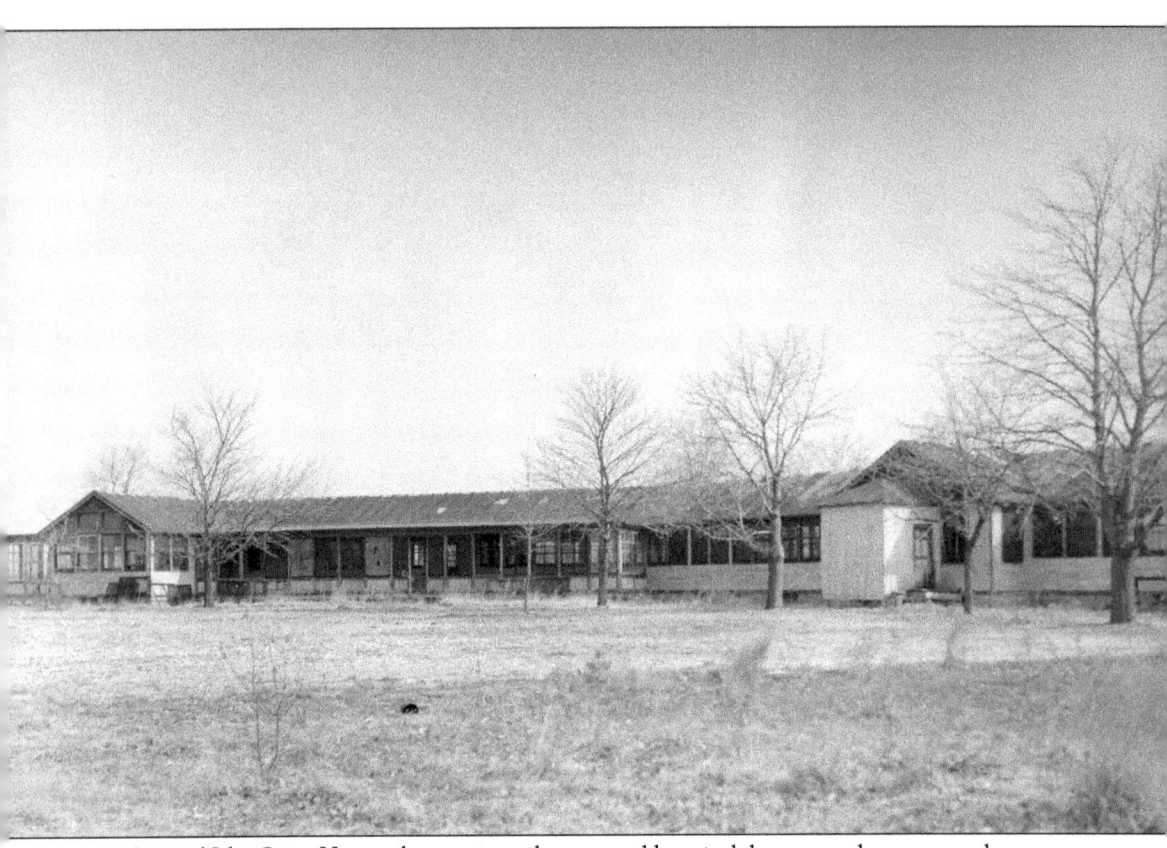

Central Islip State Hospital was primarily a mental hospital; however, there were other reasons a person could be admitted, and tuberculosis was one. A separate unit was constructed in the earlier part of the 20th century to house these patients. Due to the highly contagious nature of the disease, having a freestanding building away from the general hospital population was desirable. Until November 1949, there was no effective cure. By the 1950s, cure rates were averaging 90 percent, and tuberculosis was viewed as nearly eradicated. Due to the drastic reduction in people afflicted with the disease, the need for a separate building dwindled. This is Central Islip's tuberculosis unit in the 1960s after it closed. It was soon demolished to make way for other structures.

Two

NURSING AND MEDICAL STAFF

In the beginning at Kings Park and Central Islip, staff consisted primarily of nurses and attendants. There were few medical doctors, and virtually no other professionals to provide treatment. The ward staff, including nurses and attendants, provided 24-hour care, including patient hygiene, administering medical treatments, recreation, talk therapy, and work programs. The staff worked 12 hour days, six days a week prior to 1900. Wages were modest, with men earning $20 to $40 per month and women $14 to $18. Fringe benefits included uniforms, rubber coats & boots, food, laundry service, lodging, and a chicken and candy every Sunday. The uniform for men consisted of a navy-blue shirt and cap with a tie. For women, a blouse and long dress were worn. Men and women were to have their collars buttoned to the neck at all times while on duty, regardless of the weather. Staff arose at 5:00 a.m. to be in the hall at 5:30 to assist patients in dressing and eating breakfast. Staff lived in the halls opposite the patients and were not permitted to leave the hospital grounds at night. Watchmen patrolled the buildings and checked doors to ensure compliance. Lights were to be out for all off-duty employees at 10:30 p.m. A skeleton key inside the lock of a secured door to an employee's room was considered proof he or she was inside. Clever staff would unscrew the bars of their windows and sneak into town for a drink or smoke.

As the years went on, rules became less stringent. Shifts became eight hours and employees were allowed to leave the grounds when off duty, with the exception of young women enrolled in nursing school programs under the watch of a house mother. Attendants became known as psychiatric aides in the 1930s, and by the late 1960s, the title was again changed to mental hygiene therapy aid, or TA, as the job is known today. Nurses still provide the backbone of hospitals as providers of around-the-clock patient care.

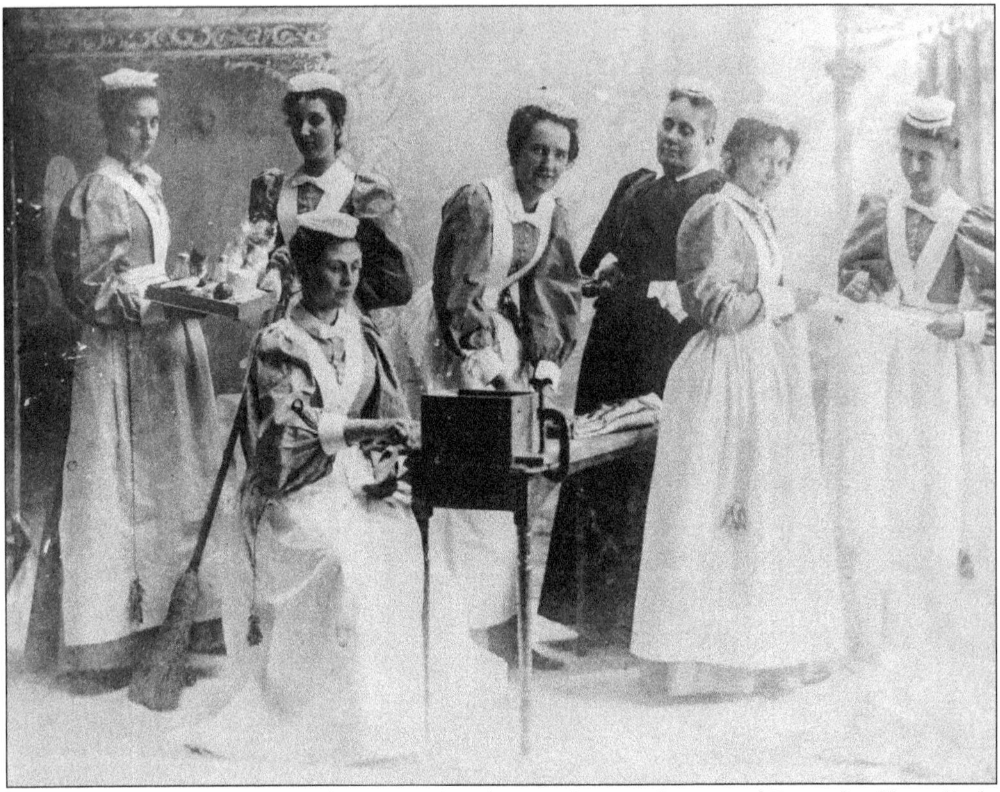

This 1890 glass-plate photograph features female attendants and nurses of Group I at Kings Park. Their uniforms were supplied at no charge by the state. Rank distinctions were determined by stripes on their caps. Navy blouses and white dresses with crossed shoulder straps were common. White bowties were worn to keep blouse collars closed while in uniform. Large keyrings can be seen hanging from the waists of the two women at right. Loss of one's keys was almost sure grounds for dismissal. When this photograph was taken, men were not permitted to work on female wards. Keys were issued to employees to match their gender. Men were forbidden to possess keys to female wards or be in female living quarters.

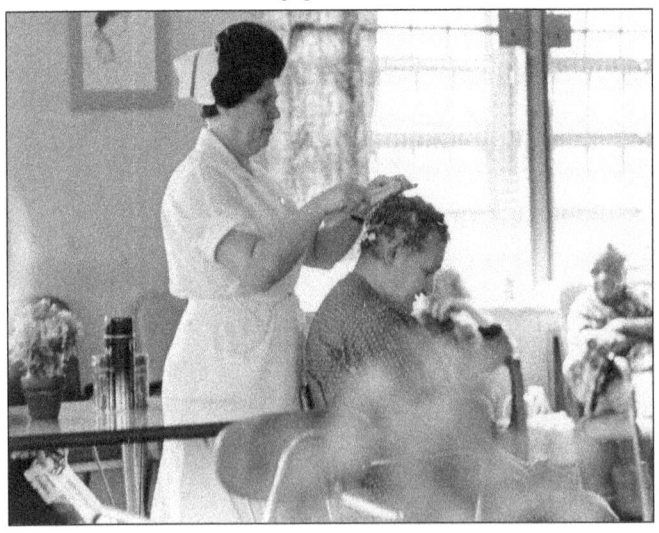

Nursing staff spent by far the most time around patients since they staffed the wards 24 hours a day, 365 days a year. As a result, they became the family many patients no longer had. Beyond their formal duties, they often took a personal interest in patients under their charge. In this 1950s image on a ward at Central Islip, a nurse is styling an older woman's hair.

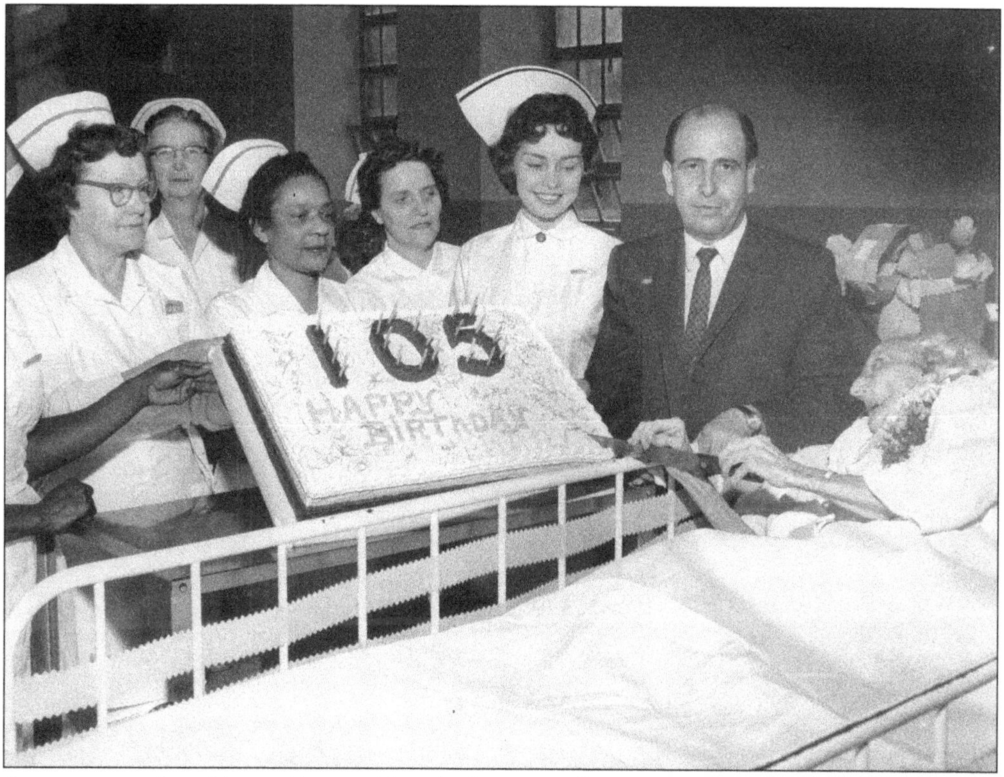

As years went by, older residents seldom had visitors. Some spent decades in the hospital and relished the opportunity to connect with the staff, volunteers, and clergy members who visited them often. Here, the nursing staff at Central Islip present a cake baked at the hospital to commemorate a woman's 105th birthday.

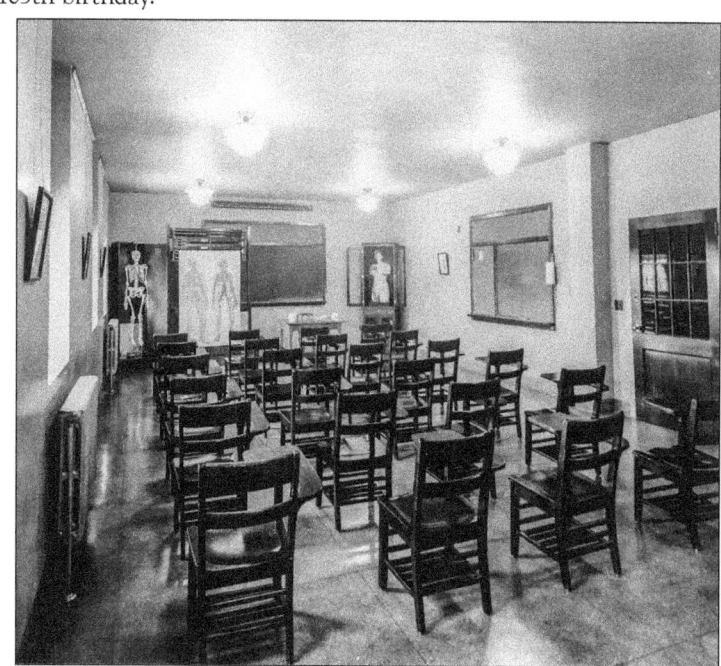

Shown here is a 1940s nursing school classroom on the upper floors of Building 23 at Pilgrim State. In the front of the classrooms were anatomical dummies for teaching purposes. Nursing school classes were smaller at the hospital than at local colleges. However, they were rigorous.

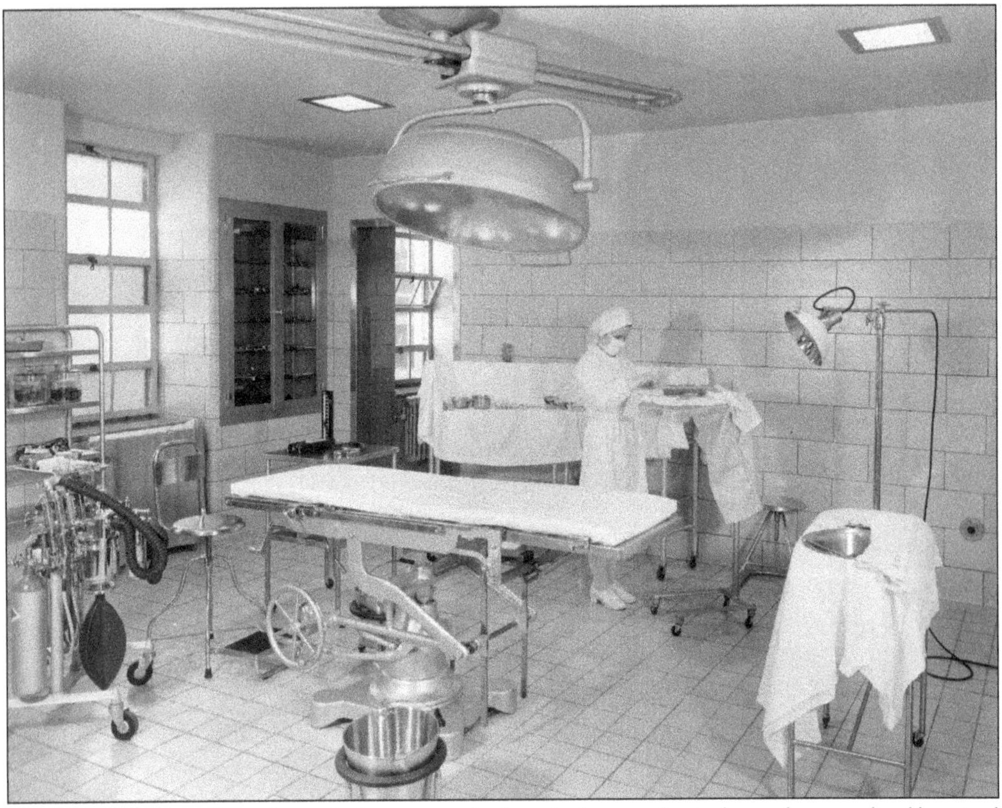

Because of the number of people living on the hospital grounds, independent medical/surgical facilities were required. As the years went on, the size and complexity of services and the level of technology increased, just as in the outside world. Here, the last operating room built on the grounds of Central Islip, in Building 126, is seen in the 1960s.

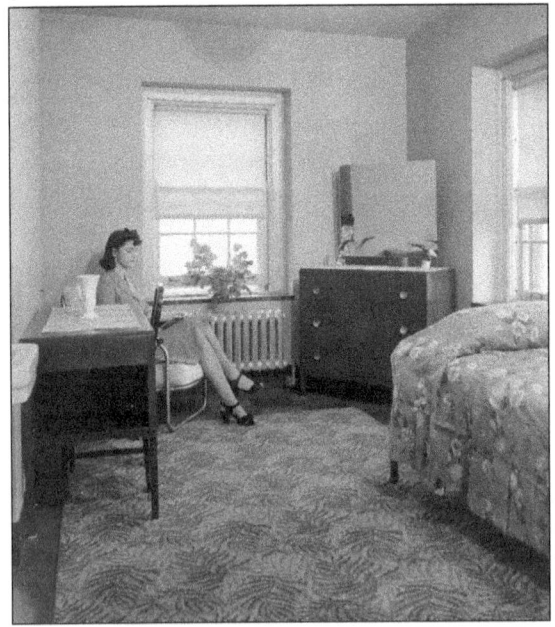

Nursing school at the state hospitals brought women, and some men, to live and work. Some students were straight out of high school, while others had previously worked as attendants at the hospital. Living on the grounds was no longer required after the turn of the 20th century; however, out of convenience or financial need, many students did. Much like a college dorm, the housing consisted of single bedrooms with a sink. Bathrooms were shared in a common area in addition to a space for socializing. This student nurse is seen during her off hours in her room at Central Islip in the 1960s.

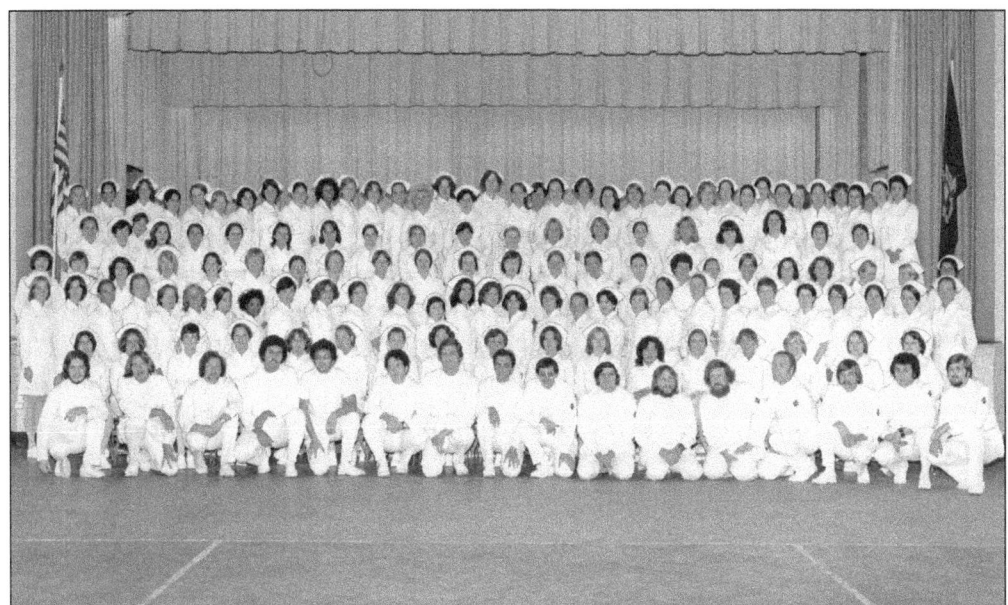

Pilgrim graduated many nurses from its nursing school. When it closed in 1978, students enrolled in the program who were halfway through the certificate were transferred to Central Islip to finish their studies. Here, the class of 1977 from Pilgrim is shown in graduation exercises with the class of 1978 at Central Islip. Third from left in the first row is Dean Weinstock, who eventually went on to be director at Pilgrim State Hospital.

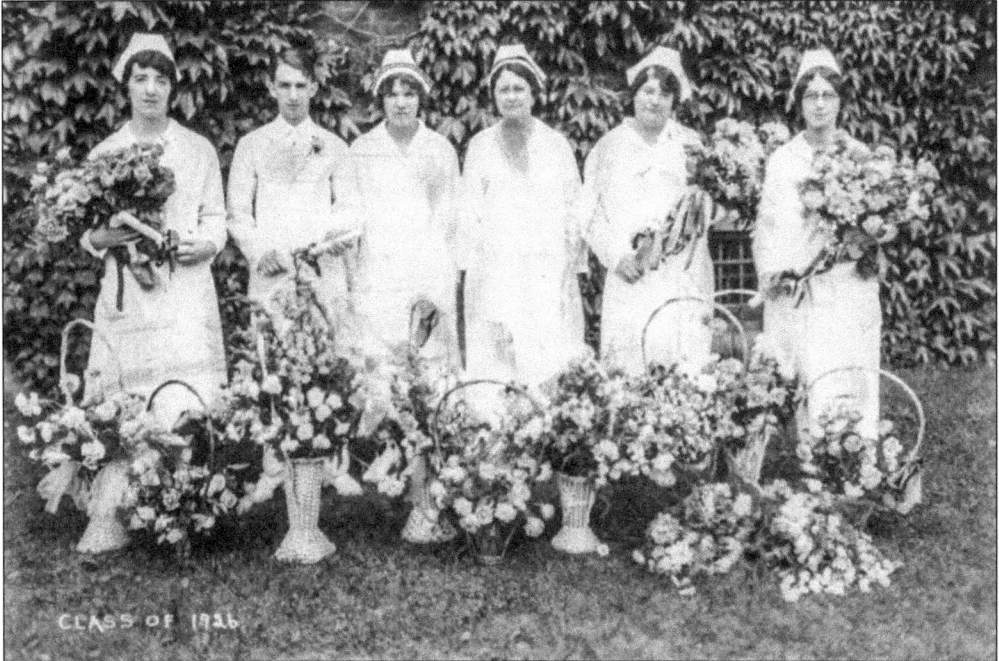

Nurses had a variety of uniforms over the decades. Employees were required to don blue and white attire. Here, at Kings Park, a group of newly graduated nurses pose in their hospital whites alongside their nurse instructors (center). Diplomas are in their hands, and their uniforms are pinned with the hospital nursing insignia. (Courtesy of the Kings Park Heritage Museum)

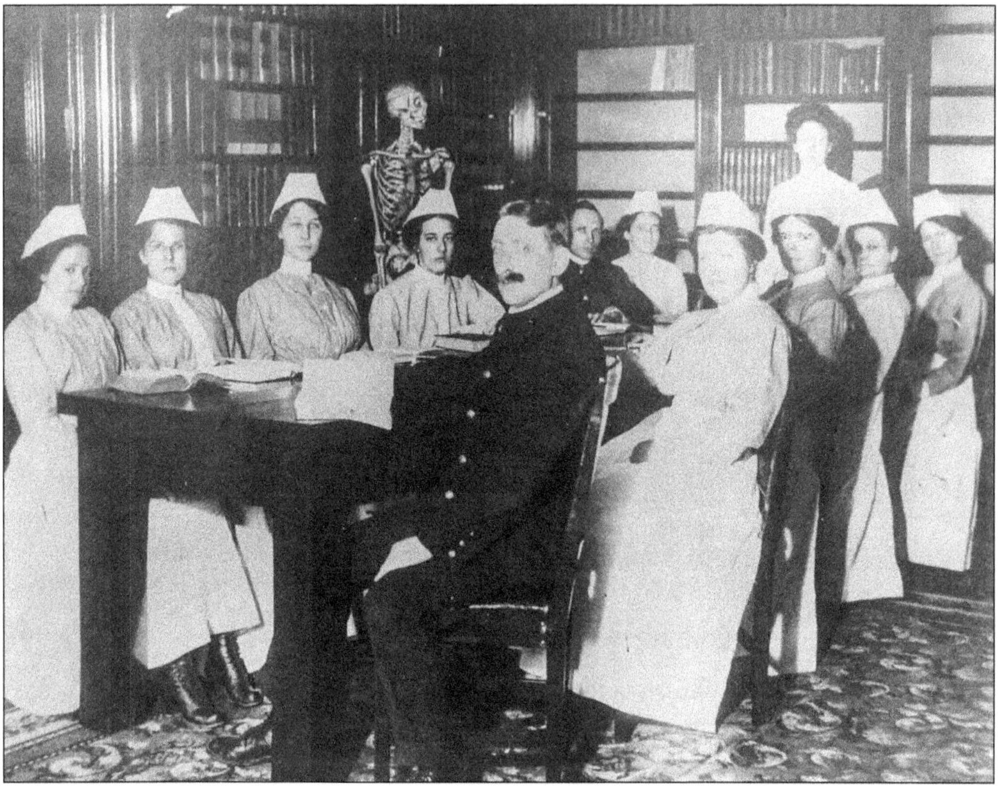

Similar to today, continuing education past college was expected of the early 20th-century nursing staff at Kings Park. This picture, taken in 1913 inside Group I, was taken during a lecture by a visiting nurse on anatomy and physiology. The men in the room, although in dark dress, were also nurses employed at the facility.

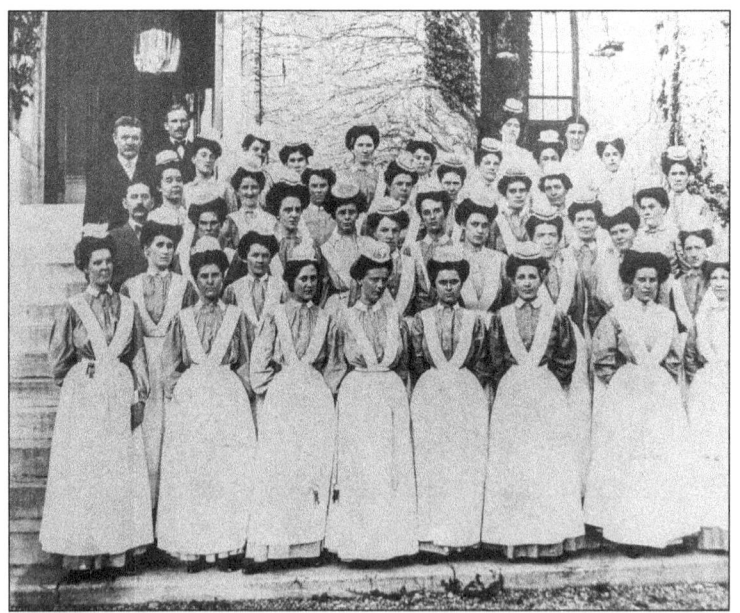

This 1890s photograph at Kings Park shows the staff nurses at the facility. Women far outnumbered men historically, although currently, the number of men in the field is increasing. These staff members posed outside of Dewing Home, an employee living quarters.

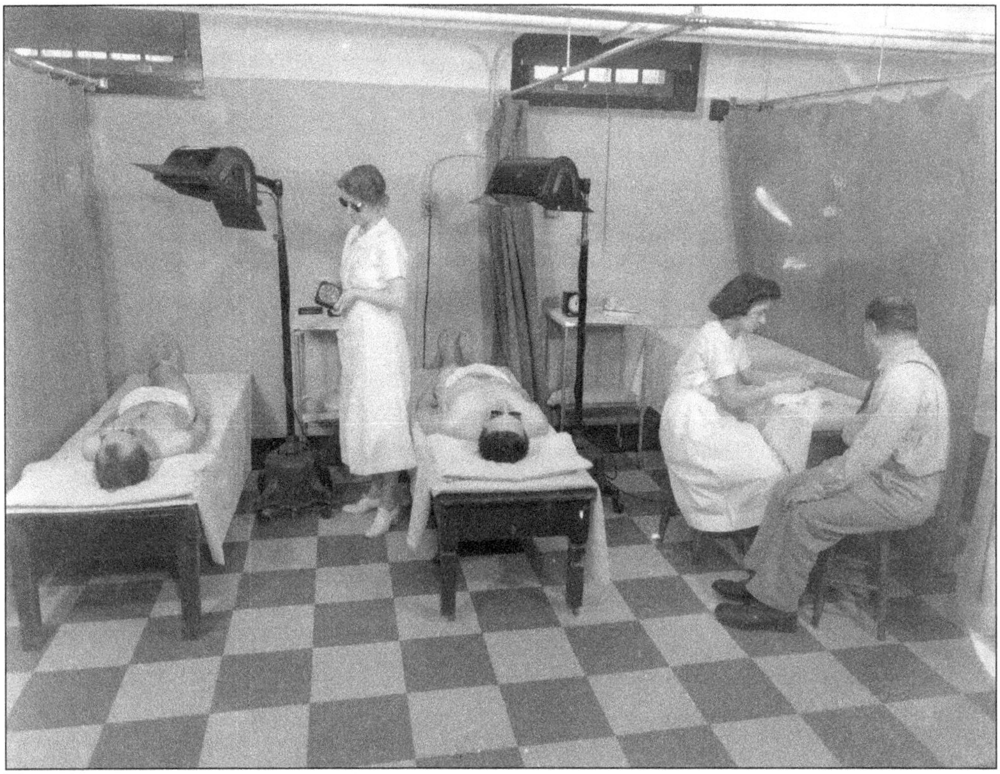

Somatic treatments have waxed and waned over the years in behavioral health. Light therapy for depression was commonplace in the 1940s when this photograph was taken at Central Islip. Patients were exposed to UV light with the intention to promote an increase in vitamin D levels. Research into light exposure for depression symptom relief is again a topic of interest among the psychiatric community.

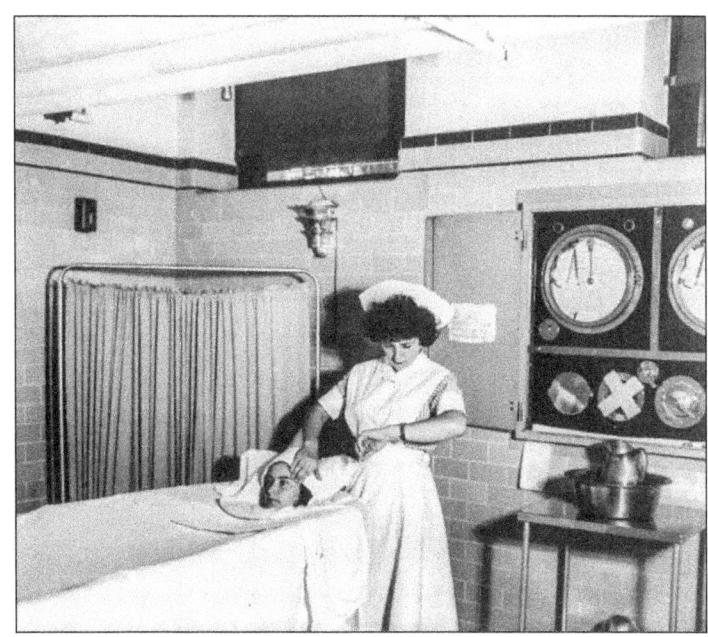

Hydrotherapy, sometimes referred to as continuous flow bath, was common in the 1950s at Central Islip. Patients were submerged in warm water to relax in order to aid in their recovery. Canvas sheets were placed over the tub to preserve modesty and trap heat. Nursing staff monitored vital signs while patients were submerged.

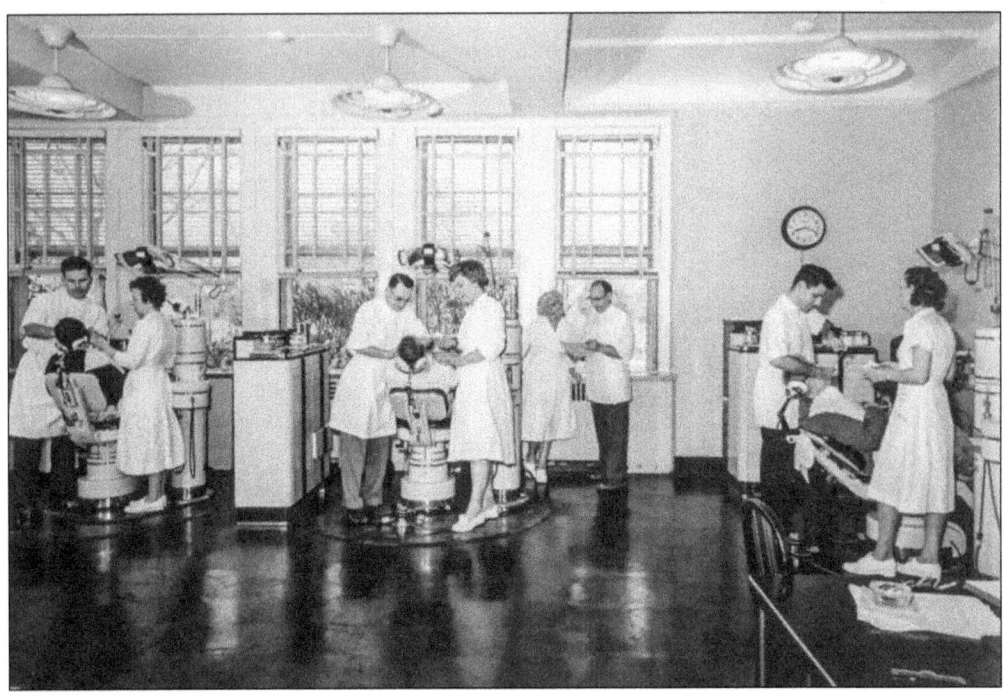

Dental clinics were a busy place at the state hospitals. Many patients, while depressed or psychotic outside the hospital, would neglect their hygiene. Any dental issues were identified during an admission examination and promptly addressed. For chronic patients living at the hospital, periodic visits for cleaning were routine. Above is the dental clinic in Building 66 at Central Islip. Building 66 was the hospital's medical/surgical services building until Building 126 was erected. Below, a similar dental clinic is shown at Edgewood State Hospital, just miles away. By providing preventive cleaning, many patients were kept safe from potentially dangerous infections. Some of them might have been unable to voice any complaints of pain or discomfort due to impairments resulting from serious mental illness.

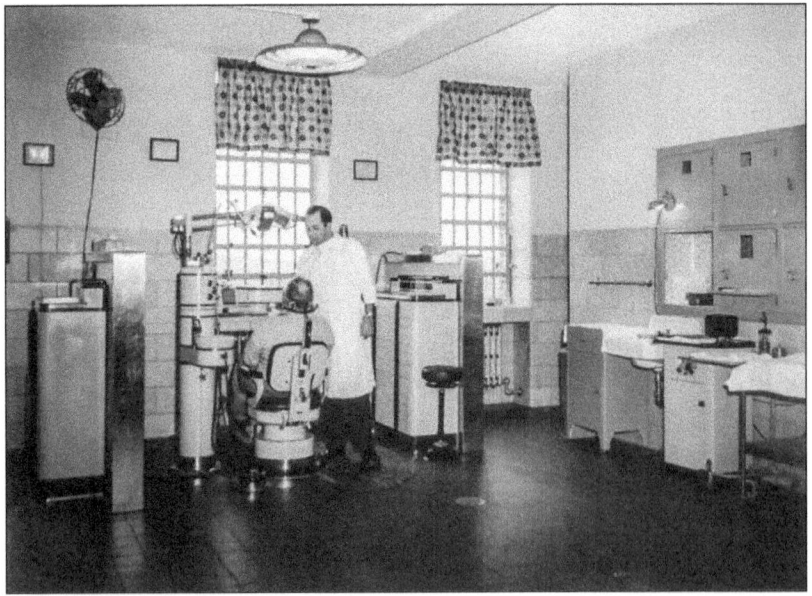

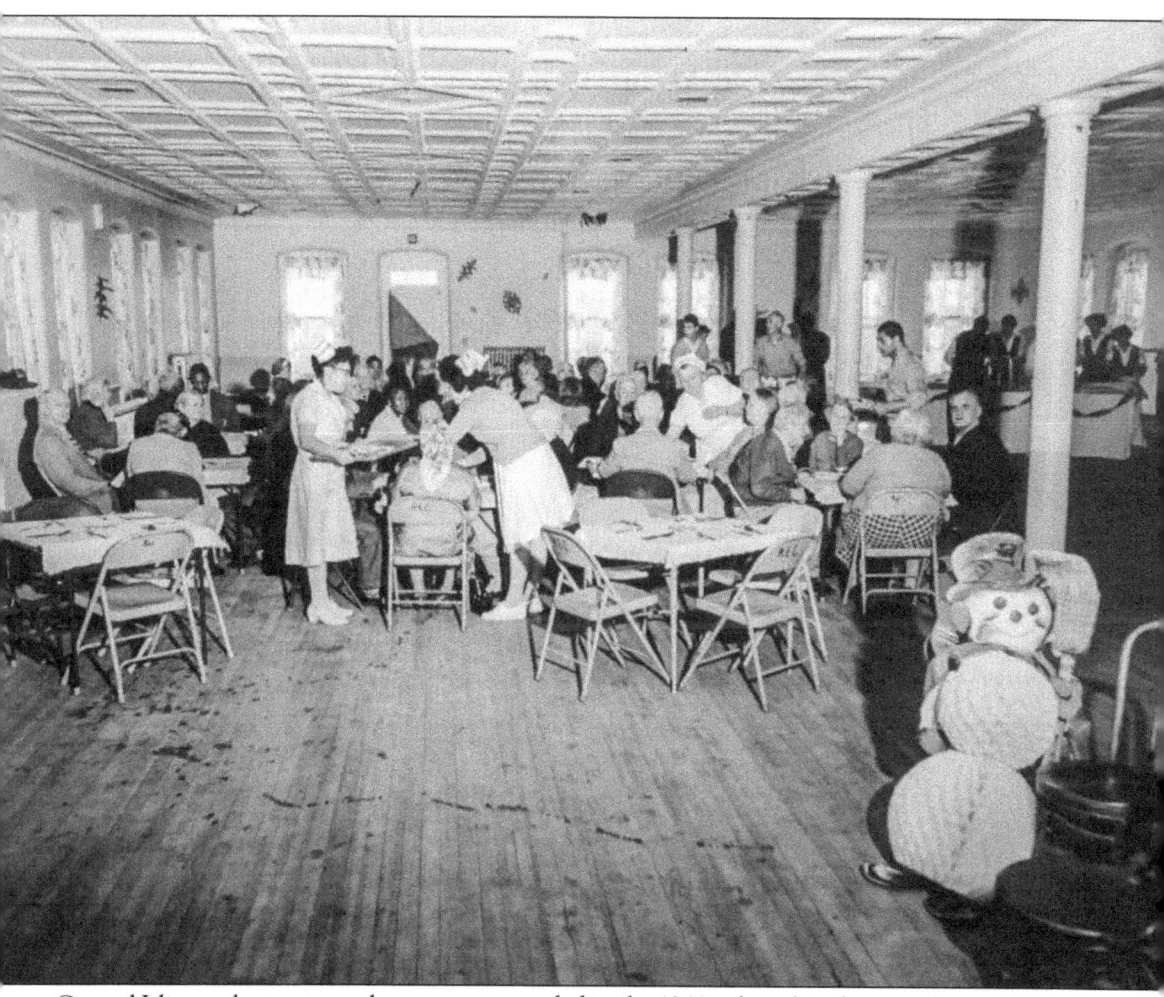

Central Islip was beginning to become overcrowded in the 1940s when this photograph was taken at the South Colony. In the coming decade, large multi-story brick buildings would replace the mostly wooden structures. The newer buildings offered greater fire protection and durability. However, mid-20th-century construction lost the aesthetically pleasing details featured in the older structures. Here, in one of the late-19th-century ward buildings, nurse aides serve a meal. In the foreground, a holiday snowman is visible. Great efforts were made by staff to make spaces feel homely and in tune with the current season. This building was one of many connected by an underground tunnel or aboveground walkway along Carleton Avenue, commonly referred to as "the String of Pearls." By the 1970s, all were vacated. Currently, modern retail stores sit on the site where these buildings were located.

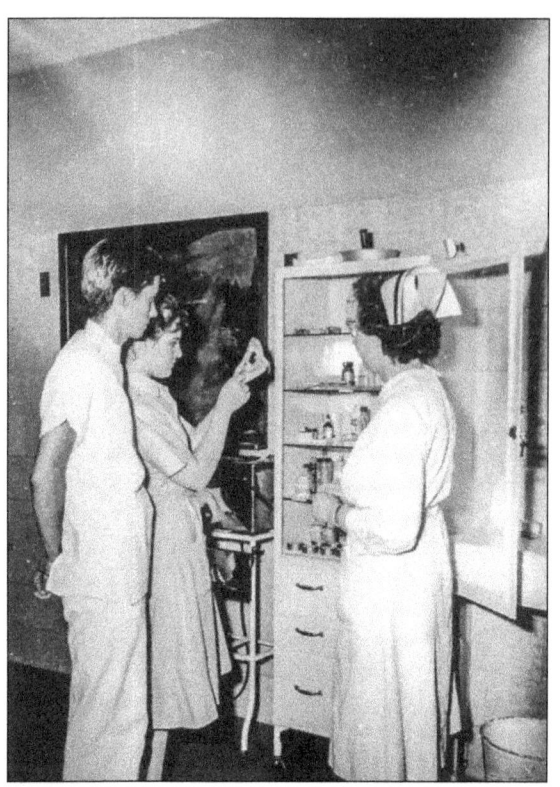

Drawing injections for everything from insulin to psychiatric medication was a daily duty for nurses at the hospital. Here, at Pilgrim State Hospital, a female student nurse takes direction from a nurse instructor. This was all part of the training program held in Building 23. A male student looks on diligently.

Administering medication to dozens of patients was one of the many tasks a nurse performed. Addressing wound care and hygienic practices were common tasks performed by most nurses as well. Here, at Pilgrim State Hospital in the 1960s, a nurse prepares a treatment for a female patient in the medical/surgical unit on the grounds.

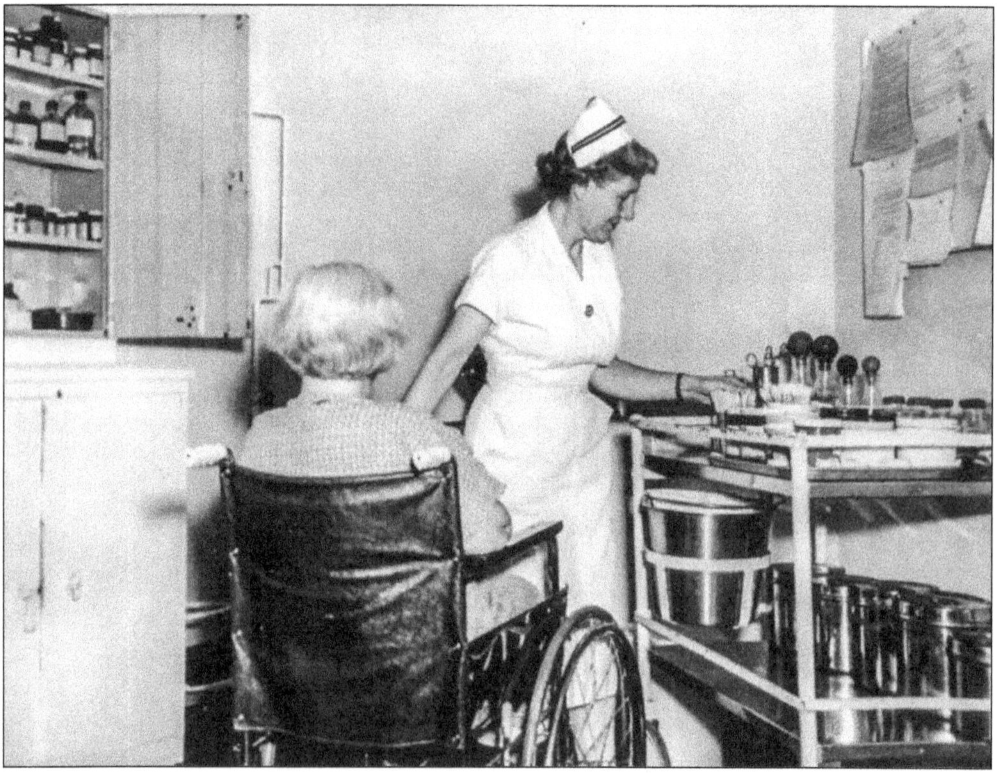

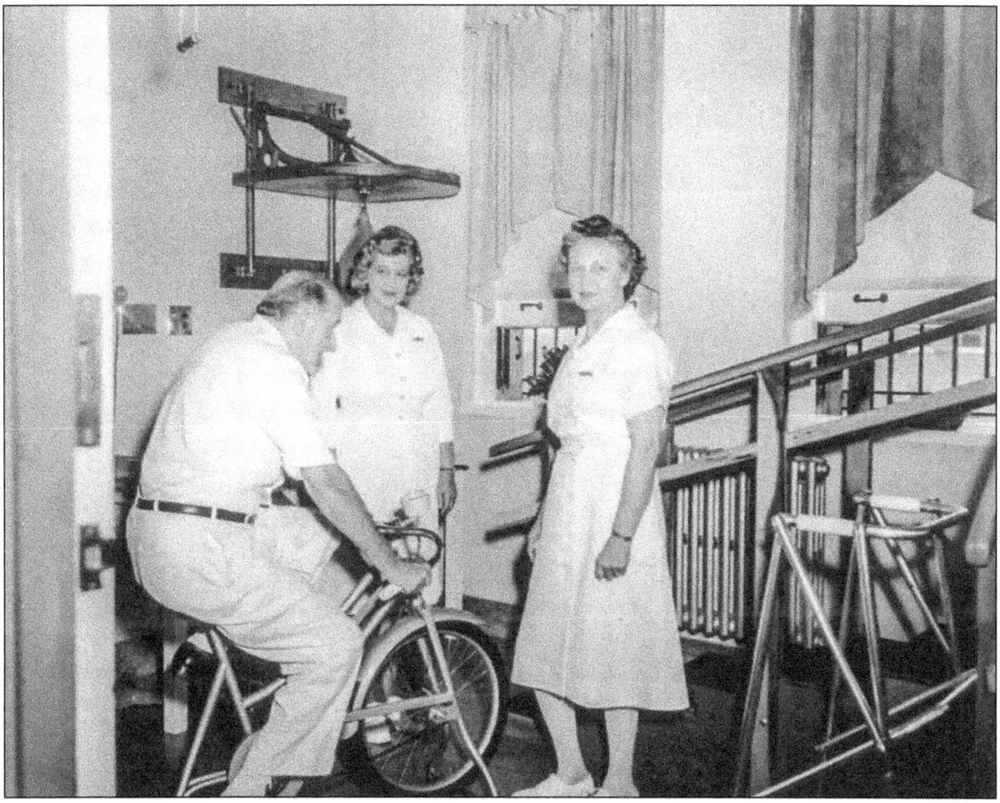

For aging individuals and those coming off bedrest for an extended period, muscle atrophy was a concern. At Central Islip, the physical therapy department provided encouragement and exercise-based therapy to help rehabilitate patients to a functional level of movement. Here, two nurses provide support to a man on an exercise bike.

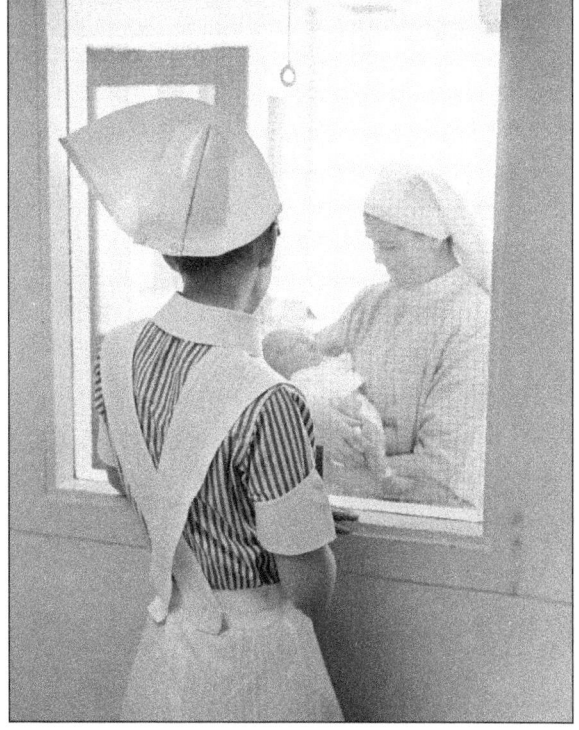

During peak operations, so many pregnant women were admitted at Central Islip that the need for its own independent maternity unit arose. Being pregnant was not viewed as a valid medical reason to be removed from a psychiatric hospital. Here, in the 1950s, a nurse looks into the neonatal unit at Central Islip. Eventually, like other medical services, this unit was transferred to the local general hospital.

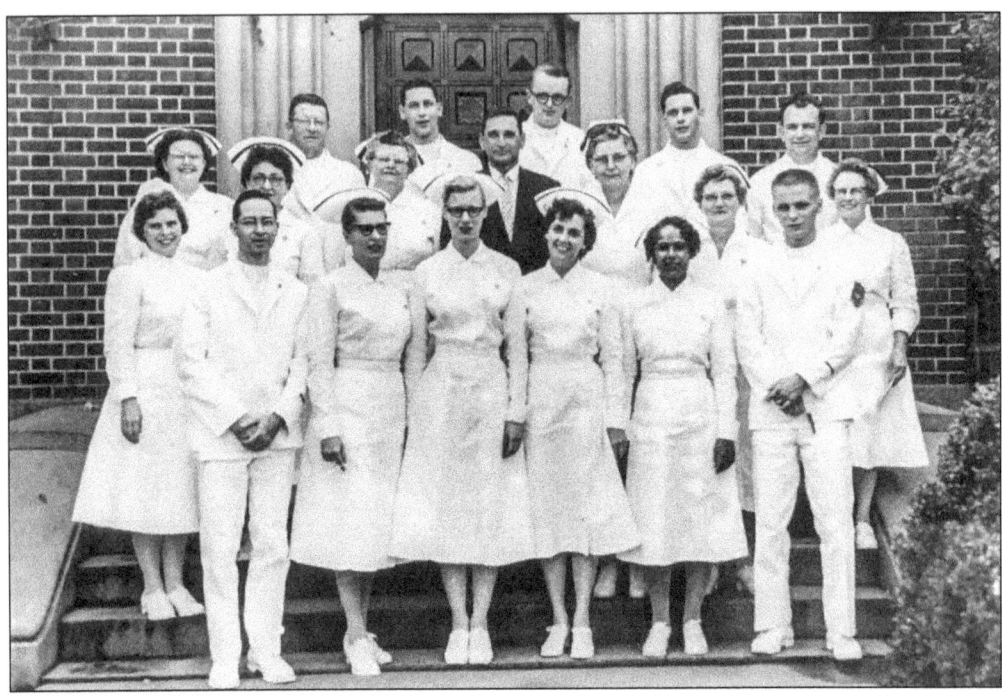

Commencement from nursing school was a happily celebrated event at the hospitals. Students waited eagerly in the assembly halls for their nursing certificate while their families, friends, and loved ones watched on from the audience. At Pilgrim State Hospital (above), a newly graduated class of nurses pose outside Building 23. Below, at Central Islip, a 1960s graduating class stands in Robbins Hall. During the ceremony, nurses were pinned with a hospital-specific nursing insignia and given a cap, as well as their certificate in nursing. Floral arrangements made at the hospital greenhouse were put on display for all attendees to enjoy.

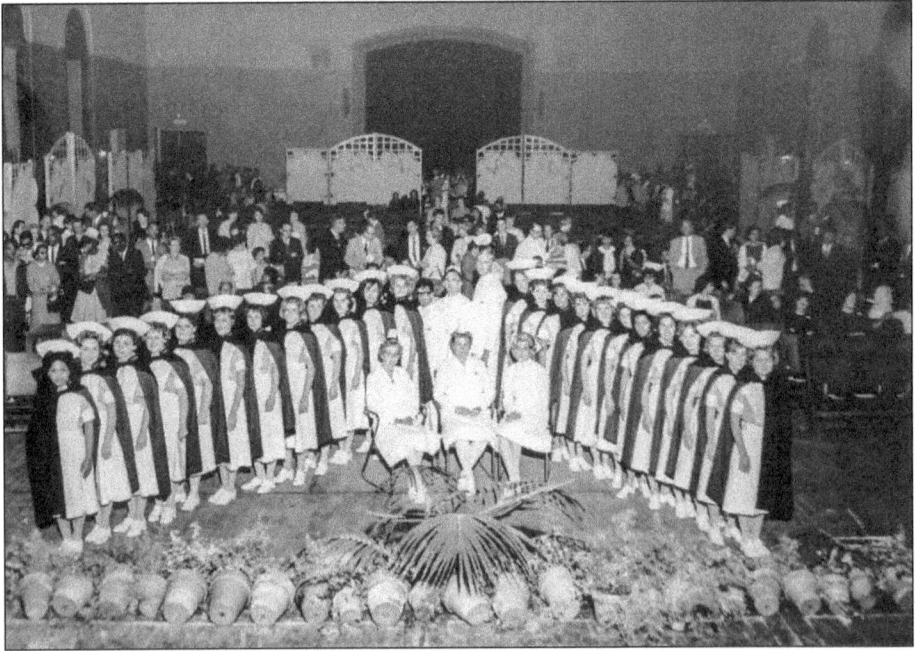

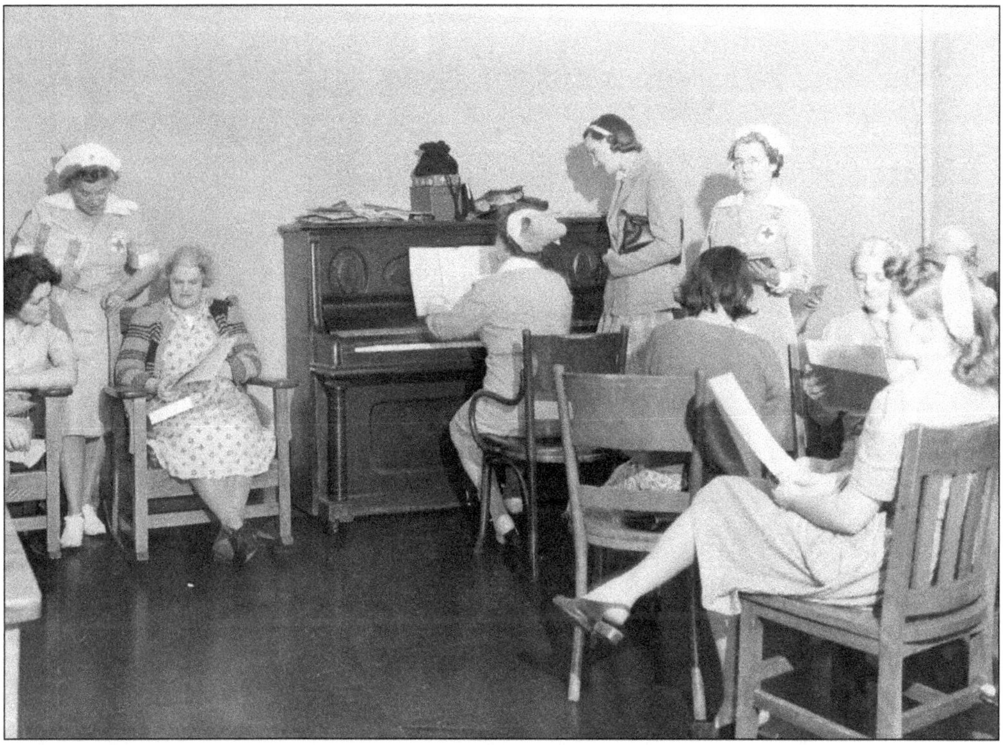

Red Cross nurses were a happy sight at the state hospitals when this photograph was taken in the 1950s. They regularly put on social events or provided companionship to patients, like the piano playing and singing shown here. Many patients were very happy to have visitors and sing along. For the patients with no visitors, the few moments of joy would provide happy reflections for weeks to come.

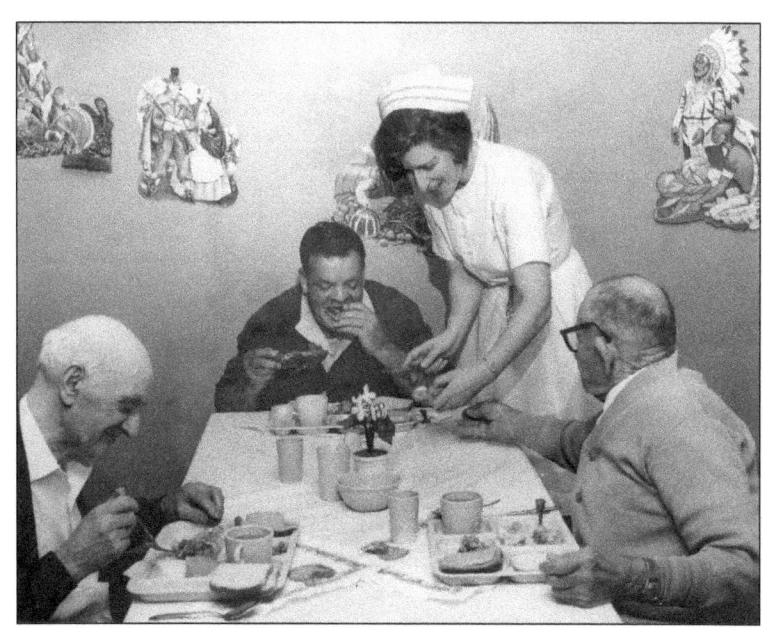

Attendants, or TAs, carried out many of the same job functions of an RN with added duties. TAs ensured that all the needs of the patients were met daily, ranging from bathing to feeding to medical attention. Here, a young TA assists men with a meal in the dining hall.

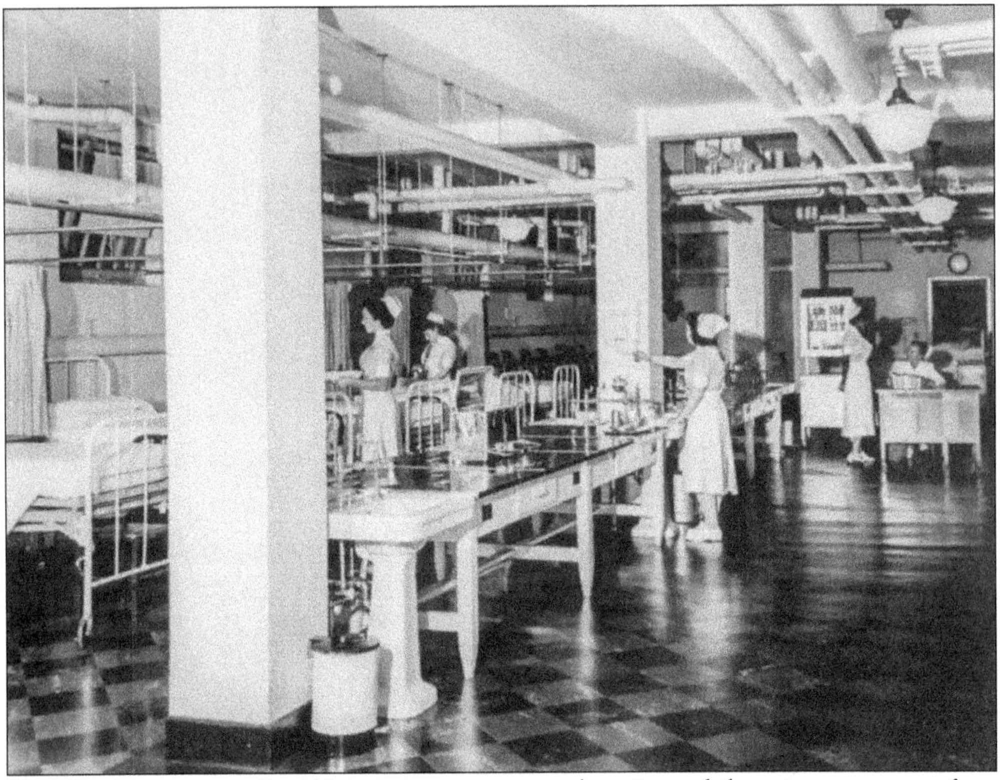

Work for the nursing staff could at times seem never-ending. Even while patients were away from the wards, there was still plenty of tasks to be completed. Here, in a medical unit at Central Islip State Hospital, nurses attend to the business of the day. Note that this unit was in a basement. Space had to be made available in creative locations to accommodate the increase in population in the 1950s.

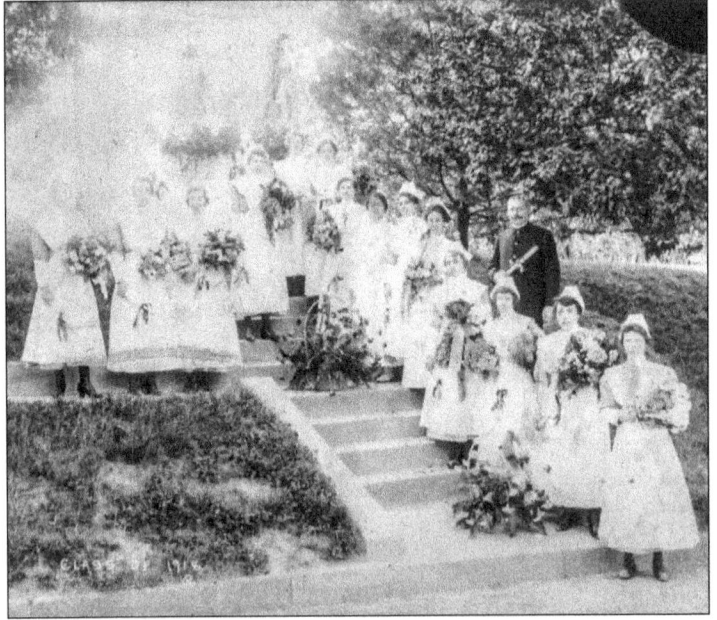

Glass-plate negatives create a very distinctive print. Although damaged by age and environment, this glass plate offers a sharp look at the graduating nursing class of 1918 at Kings Park. Nurses hold their newly received certificate and flowers to commemorate the event. At right, a man in dark attire holds his certificate proudly. (Courtesy of the Kings Park Heritage Museum.)

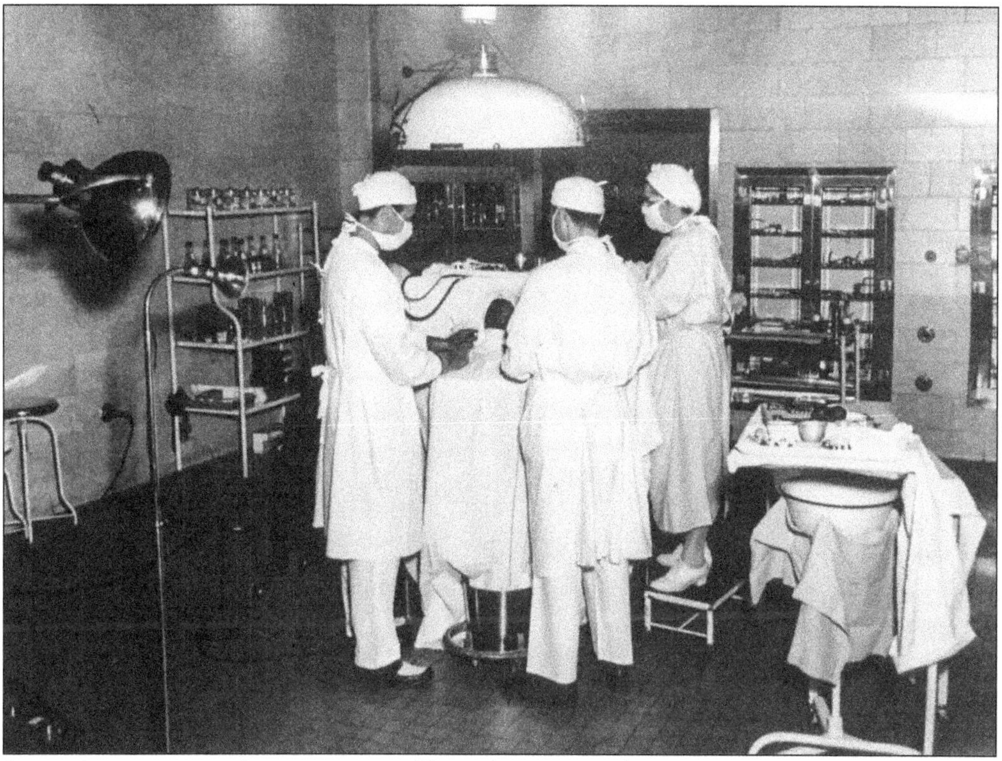

Surgical services were for many years addressed onsite at Pilgrim State Hospital in Building 23. By the 1990s, the center was no longer performing major surgeries. Here, in a 1950s photograph, surgeons prepare to operate. Typically, nurses were also assigned to the ER to assist during procedures as well as in preparatory and aftercare work.

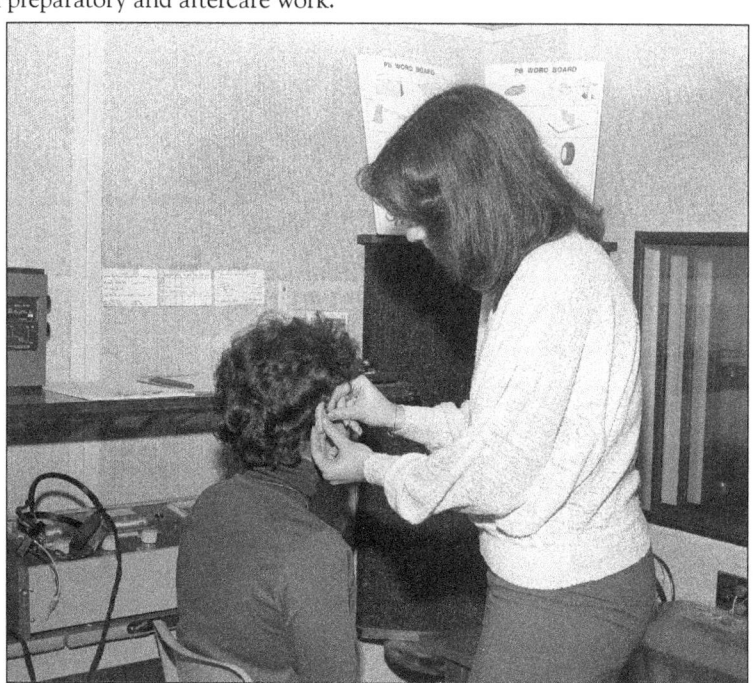

Hearing and vision were two other faculties assessed upon admission. Here, an audiological worker fits a woman for a hearing aid. After determining size, functioning of the device was also tested at the clinic. The hearing clinic, like most clinics, was in the medical service building at Pilgrim State Hospital.

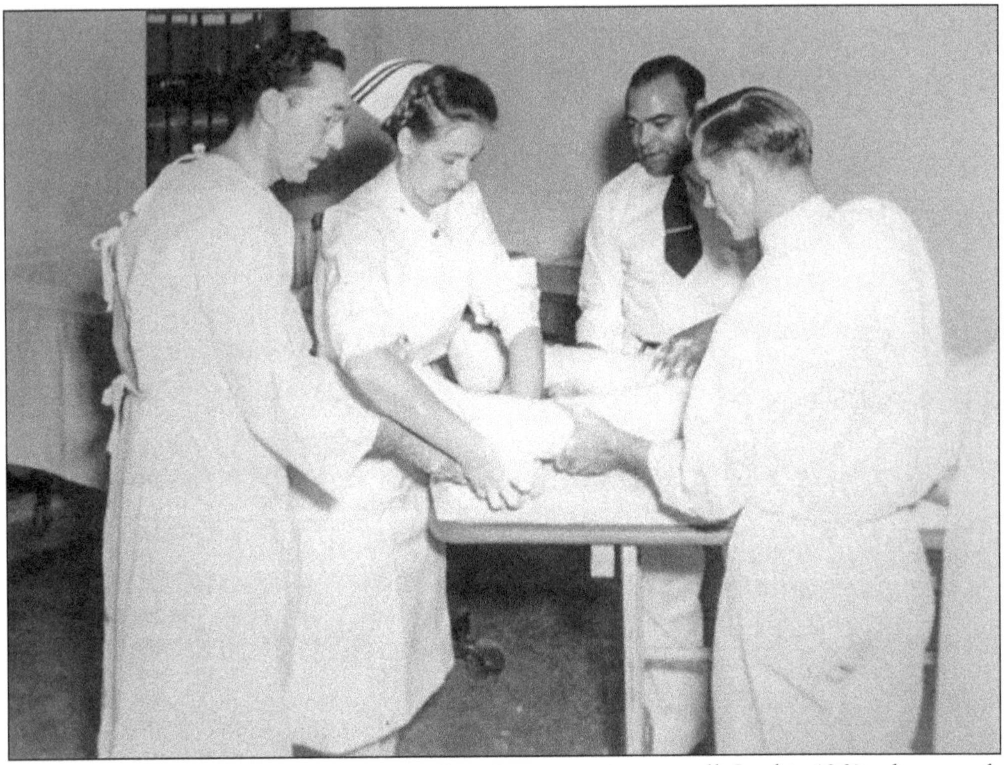

Injuries that required casting were treated at the institution as well. In this 1960s photograph taken at the hospital clinic at Edgewood, a physician, nurse, and attendants work together to apply a cast to a patient. Addressing medical complications onsite allowed the patients to be treated by staff they knew well instead of strangers at a local hospital.

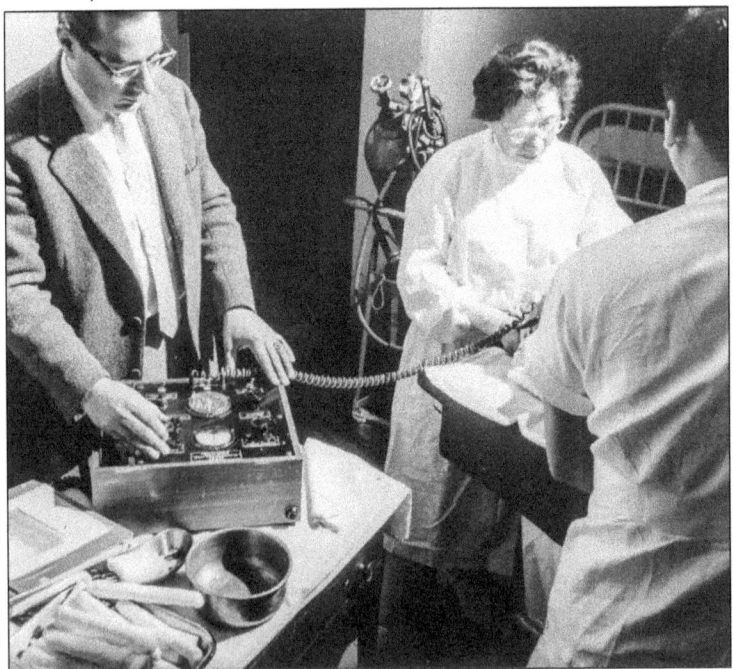

Electroconvulsive Therapy (ECT) is often misrepresented. This treatment is used only in the most extreme cases, after all other options are exhausted. ECT has been largely effective in depression treatment for those who do not respond well to drug therapy. This photograph was taken in the 1930s during an ECT treatment in Building 66, the medical/surgical services unit of Central Islip State Hospital.

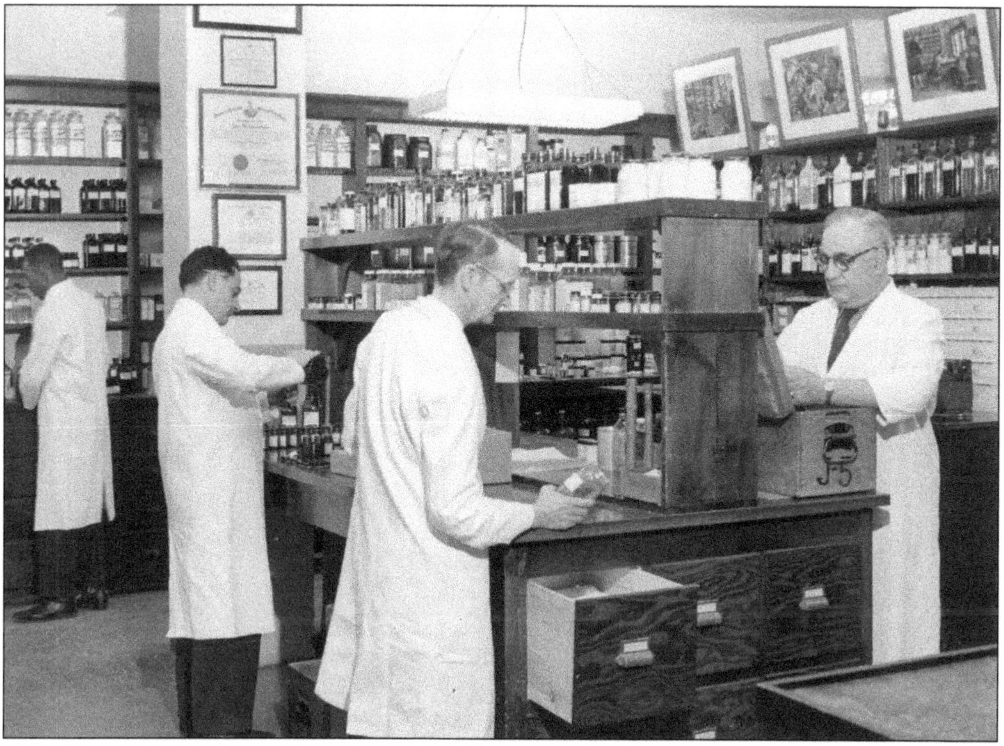

The pharmacy at each state hospital produced a massive amount of tonics, ointments, and other prescriptions. Until the 1990s, each facility still compounded certain medications onsite. Above, the pharmacy at Central Islip is pictured in the 1950s. Shelves full of chemicals used to make medication are visible. To the right is a wooden box marked "J-5." Boxes like this were filled with medicine and locked at the pharmacy, then returned to the nurse on the ward, who had a key to unlock it. Below, at Pilgrim State's pharmacy in the late 1960s, a board of such keys hangs in front of a pharmacy staff member.

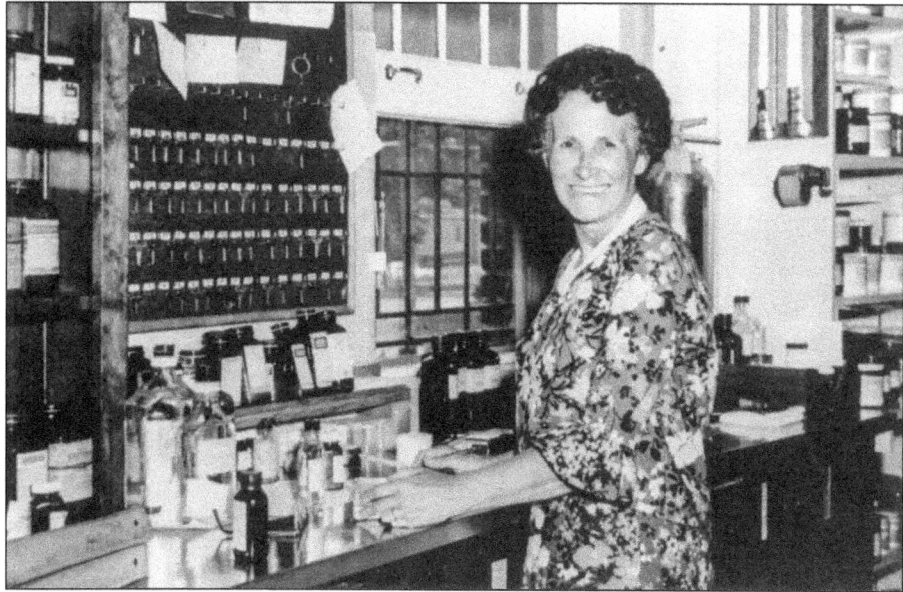

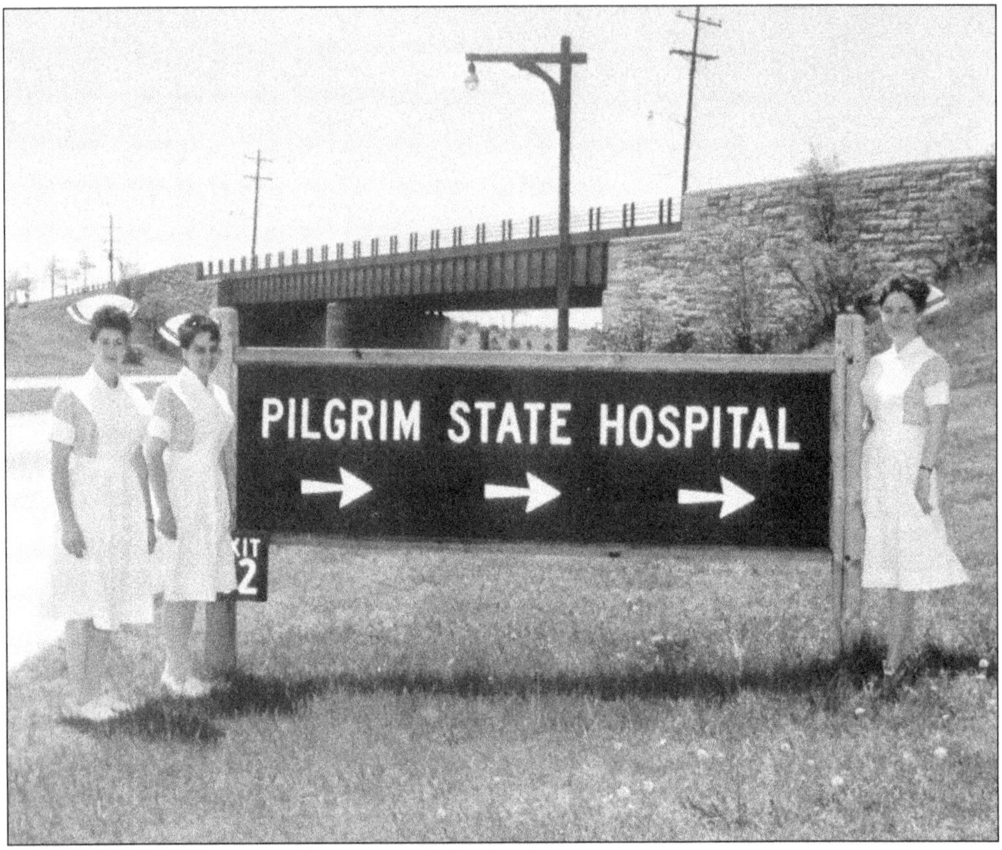

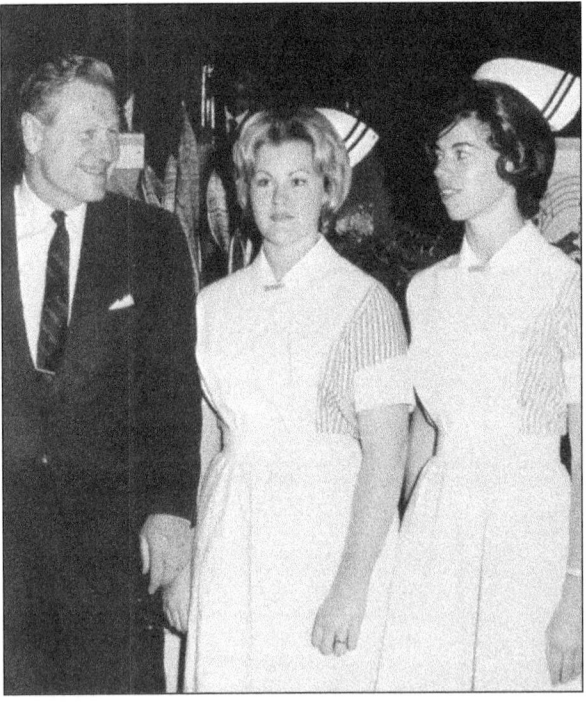

For many, attending nursing school at the state hospitals was a very memorable experience. Students often came straight out of high school from diverse areas. The nursing programs were attractive because of affordability as well as the opportunity to attend school, live in a dormitory, and rotate to several institutions around downstate New York for fieldwork. Above, student nurses pose with the entrance sign to Pilgrim State Hospital in the 1960s. A close look at their caps reveals vertical stripes on the right side, different from the horizontal stripe of a graduate RN cap. This was to distinguish students and identify how far along in training they were. At left, two student RNs from Pilgrim State pose with Governor Rockefeller while completing their field training at the Willowbrook State School.

Three

FIRE, POLICE, AND WARTIME

Like a small town, the state hospitals required independent services to fight fires due to their remote locations. In the pioneer days, men manned bucket brigades with few tools and equipment. In 1903, the old laundry building at Central Islip State Hospital was retrofitted to accommodate 14 men who acted as firemen. The building was initially equipped with a horse-drawn carriage, hooks and ladders, and other hand tools. The fire department at Central Islip was officially organized in 1907, with 10 employees volunteering under a retired New York City Fire Department lieutenant. James Maloney, who worked in the power plant, served as chief. Under Chief Maloney, the firemen trained to dress quickly and slide down a pole from their quarters into the engine room, to arrive at their post as fast as possible after an alarm was received. Hospital watchmen were tasked with duties typically associated with policemen of the time, with additional emphasis on enforcing staff regulations in the early days. Watchmen were additionally charged with preserving good order in the hospital, with foot patrols recorded in the supervisor's office by the turn of a watch-clock key.

Kings Park State Hospital underwent growth equivalent to Central Islip, requiring independent fire and police services. Close to 900 acres of property were occupied by Kings Park. Primarily consisting of wooden buildings and virtually no uniform building codes, fire was a reality that could prove deadly without fast action. As the fire and law enforcement services grew independently, the safety department was the resulting combination of both services on the hospital grounds. In 1973, safety officers began issuing summons answerable to Suffolk County Court, replacing tickets answered at the hospital. In 1931, Pilgrim State Hospital was surrounded by an expanse of scrub oak and stunted pine trees in a sandy plain. With passing time, towns sprung up and formed municipal fire departments. The title of safety officer came to be primarily a law enforcement position combined with fire prevention by the 1980s, as it largely remains today.

CENTRAL ISLIP STATE HOSPITAL
SYSTEM OF FIRE SIGNALS
FIRE ALARM BOX NUMBERS AND LOCATIONS

SOUTH COLONY		NORTH COLONY	
NUMBER OF BOX	LOCATION	NUMBER OF BOX	LOCATION
1.1.2	K-5	1.3.8	Hoffman House
1.1.3	K Center	1.3.9	Administration Building
1.1.4	K-2	2.2.2	S-5
1.1.5	I-3	2.2.3	S Kitchen
1.1.6	I-2	2.2.4	S-2
1.1.7	Print Shop, I-5 & Laundry	2.2.5	North Colony Staff House
1.1.8	South Colony Power House	2.2.6	M Group
1.2.2	H-3	Telephone	A Group
1.2.3	H-2		B Group
1.2.4	G-3	Telephone	HOME 5
1.2.5	G-2	2.2.9	Bakery
1.2.6	G Home	2.3.3	Officers' Cottages 1 to 7 Inclusive
1.2.7	H-5, H-6 & H Linen Room	2.3.4	Senior Director's Residence
1.3.4	J Building	2.4.4	F Group
1.3.5	Mills Home	2.4.5	E Group
1.3.6	Viele Home	2.4.6	D 4, 5, 6
	Maintenance Shops	2.4.7	D 1, 2, 3
	Robbins Hall	2.4.8	North Colony Home
	Infirmary Building 95	2.4.9	Garage
	L-1, 2, & 3	2.5.6	FIRE HOUSE
	L-4, 5 & 6	2.5.7	Stables and Sheds
Telephone	Admission Service	2.5.8	Cow Barn
	L Dining Room & Kitchen		Chicken Yard
	Homes 1, 2, 3, 4	Telephone	Piggery
	Officers' Apartment Houses A, B, C		Shoe Shop
	Officers' Apartment House 88		

Fire Gongs and Registers will Strike Off the Numbers

In case of fire at any of these districts, an alarm should be given only from fire box in district where fire is located, by pulling the handle and then pulling down the lever; also telephone to the main office. (Other boxes in other districts should not be disturbed if there is no fire in that district.)

In case of fire at night first give the still alarm, which is by telephone; if that fails, give general alarm if the fire gets beyond your control.

The sight of smoke or the smell of burning material is sufficient cause to give a still alarm.

No confusion or cry of fire should be given, but if at night, call all employees sleeping in the building where the fire is detected.

Everybody must respond to a fire call. In case of fire at the North Colony, those in the South Colony shall remain in the South Colony and vice versa, but in all cases of alarm, everybody should go on duty to their separate wards, and wait for instructions.

All employees not connected with the ward service are to respond immediately to the place of the fire, night or day.

The siren will signal one (1) for the North Colony with intervals and two (2) for the South Colony with intervals. The siren will not be used at night except in emergency and by instruction

DAVID CORCORAN, M.D., SENIOR DIRECTOR

The advent of the telegraph was not only a revolution in communication for the professional world, but for the fire service as well. Alarms once sounded by whistle or bell were now able to be tripped by the pull of a mechanism that would send out a preprogrammed message in Morse code to a central station in the firehouse. The sound produced when the keys struck the paper eventually became known as "mark and space," an inkless tapping of keys recorded by the telegraph receiver. The alarm was locally known as a gong because of the sound the audible alarm in the building made. When the alarm was pulled in the building, the pull station could not be reset until a fireman responded and inserted a key. At the firehouse, the receiving mechanism for the telegraph printed out a small paper recording the location of the alarm.

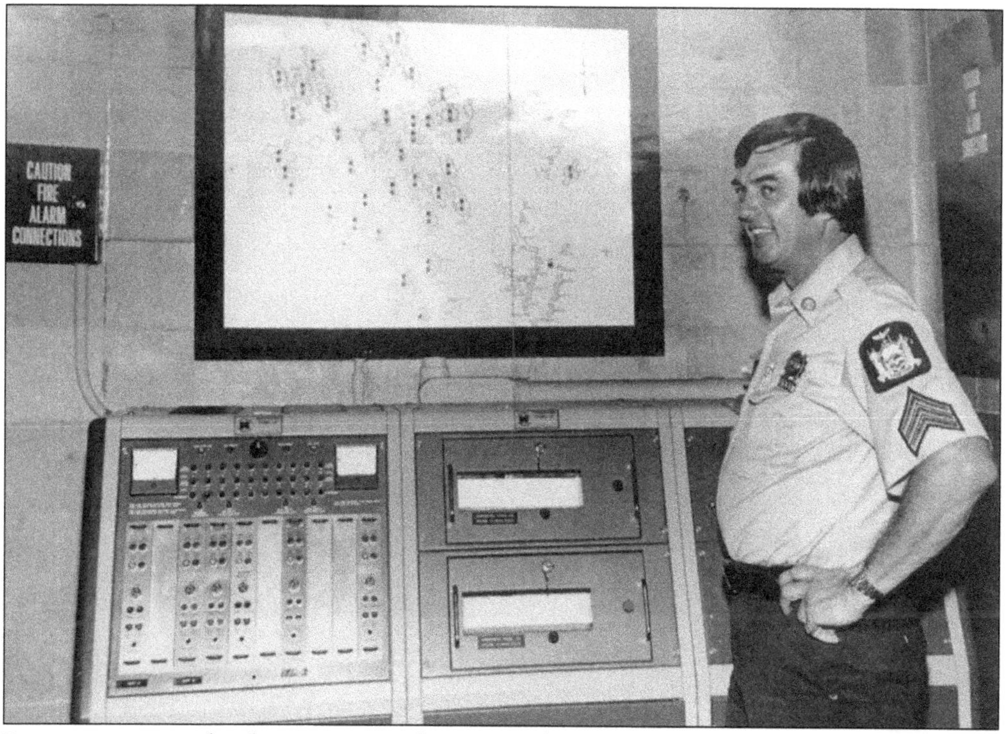

Fire monitoring technology grew over the years to become more sophisticated. With dozens of buildings on a 1,800-acre wooded expanse at Pilgrim State Hospital, speedy fire response was most certainly a vital function. In this 1960s image, Sgt. Roy DuJat can be seen near the alarm panel at Pilgrim State Hospital. A map of the grounds with each building can be seen.

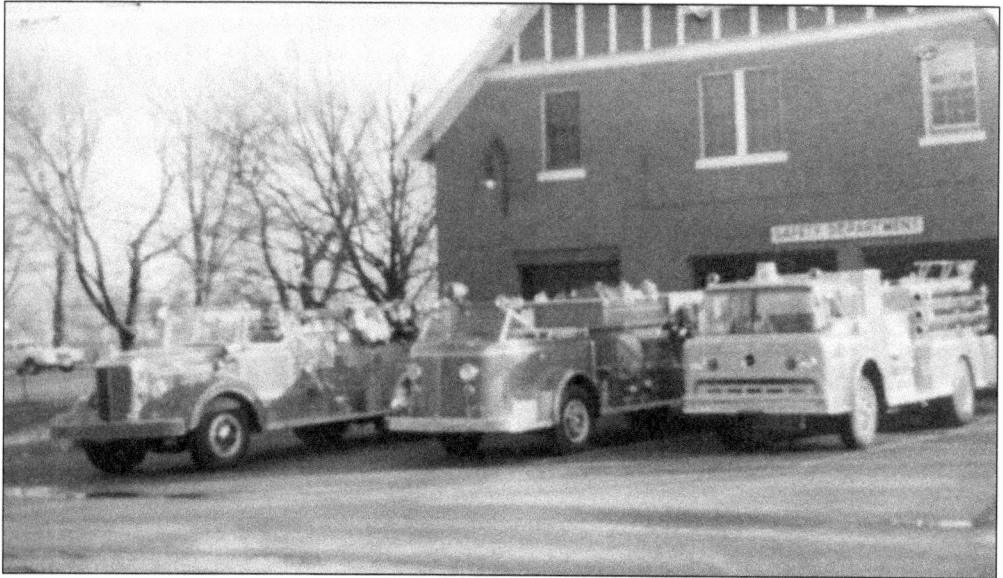

Much progress was made at the Central Islip State Hospital Fire Department since its beginnings in 1907. The horse-drawn pumps were replaced with motorized engines as they became commercially available. In this 1970s image, an older engine is at left, with the firefighters' turnout gear hanging on the back. To the right is the newer Mack fire engine.

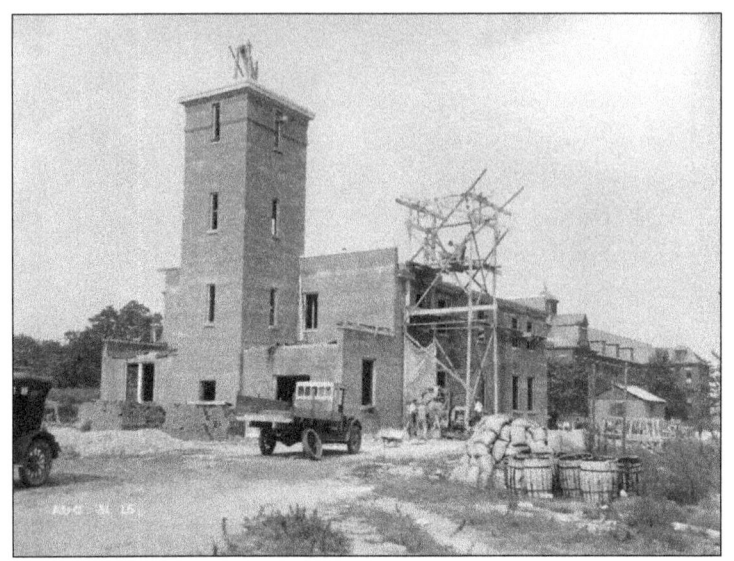

In 1925, construction was underway at Kings Park State Hospital for a state-of-the-art brick firehouse. In this image, the progress of the building's construction can be seen. The tall tower to the rear was for hanging wet hoses to dry. In those days, hoses were made of cloth and were susceptible to rot if not properly dried.

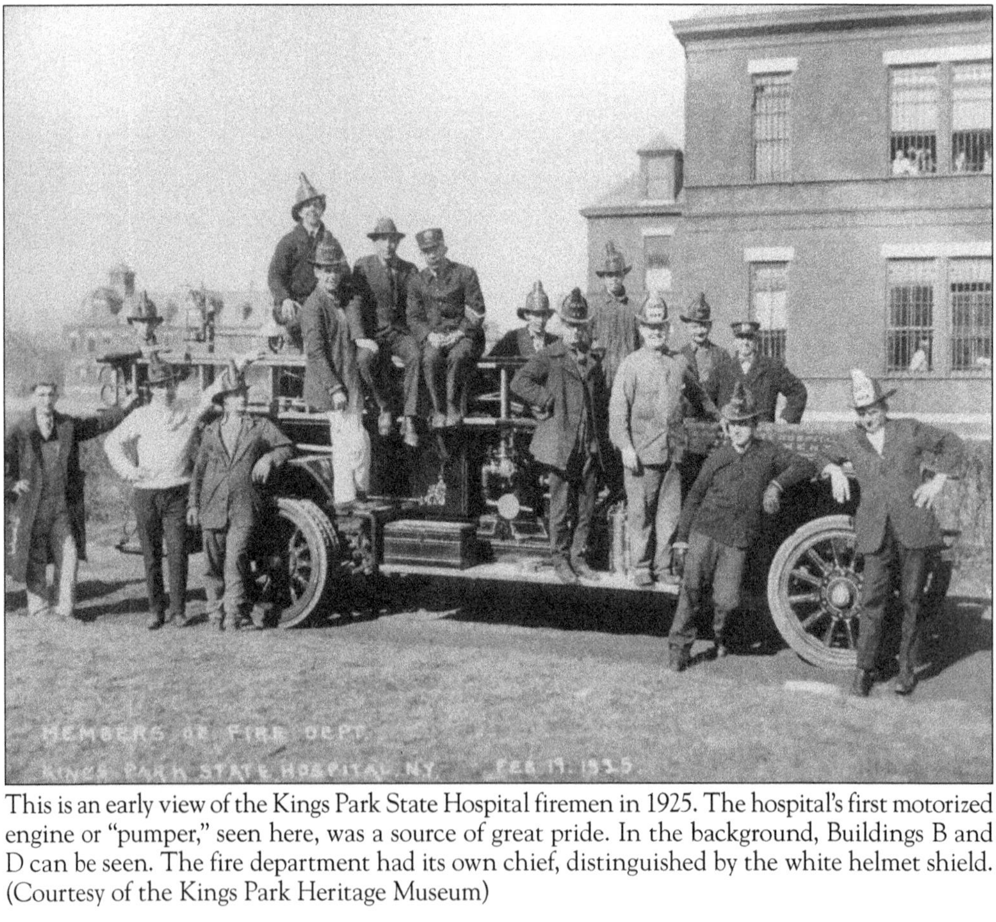

This is an early view of the Kings Park State Hospital firemen in 1925. The hospital's first motorized engine or "pumper," seen here, was a source of great pride. In the background, Buildings B and D can be seen. The fire department had its own chief, distinguished by the white helmet shield. (Courtesy of the Kings Park Heritage Museum.)

Holding drills to keep firemen's skills sharp has been a long-standing tradition. Here, in the 1960s at Pilgrim State Hospital, members of the fire department get ready to perform a pumping drill in a field. The helmets and boots worn by the firemen of that time can be seen on the truck. "Irons," or the ax and Halligan bar, still in use today, were mounted on the truck's rear.

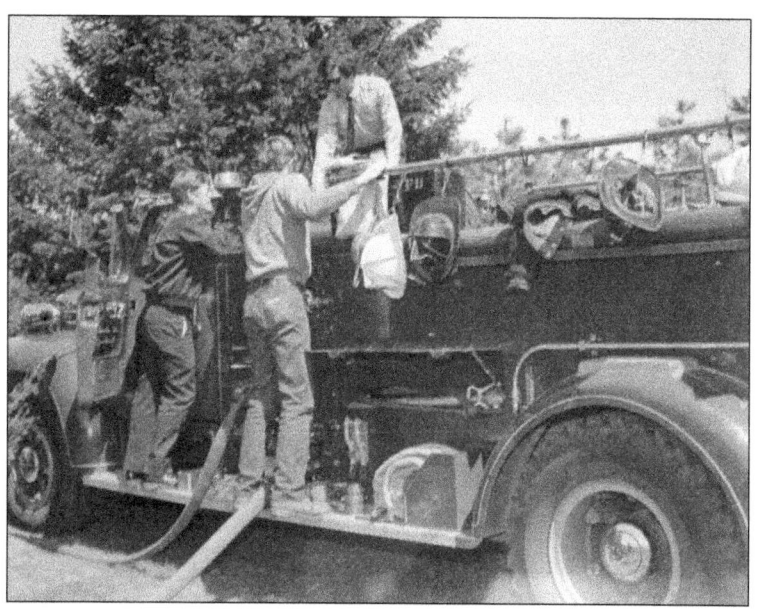

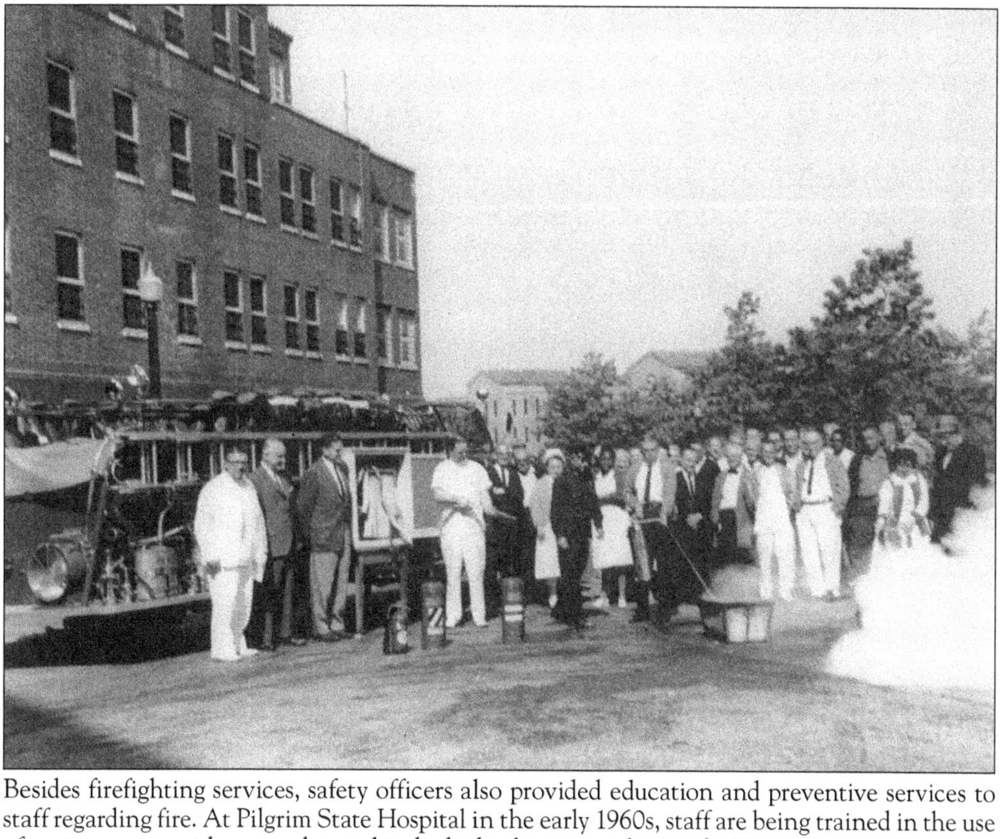

Besides firefighting services, safety officers also provided education and preventive services to staff regarding fire. At Pilgrim State Hospital in the early 1960s, staff are being trained in the use of various extinguisher cans located in locked cabinets on the wards. Fire prevention days were held annually for many years at all of the state hospitals.

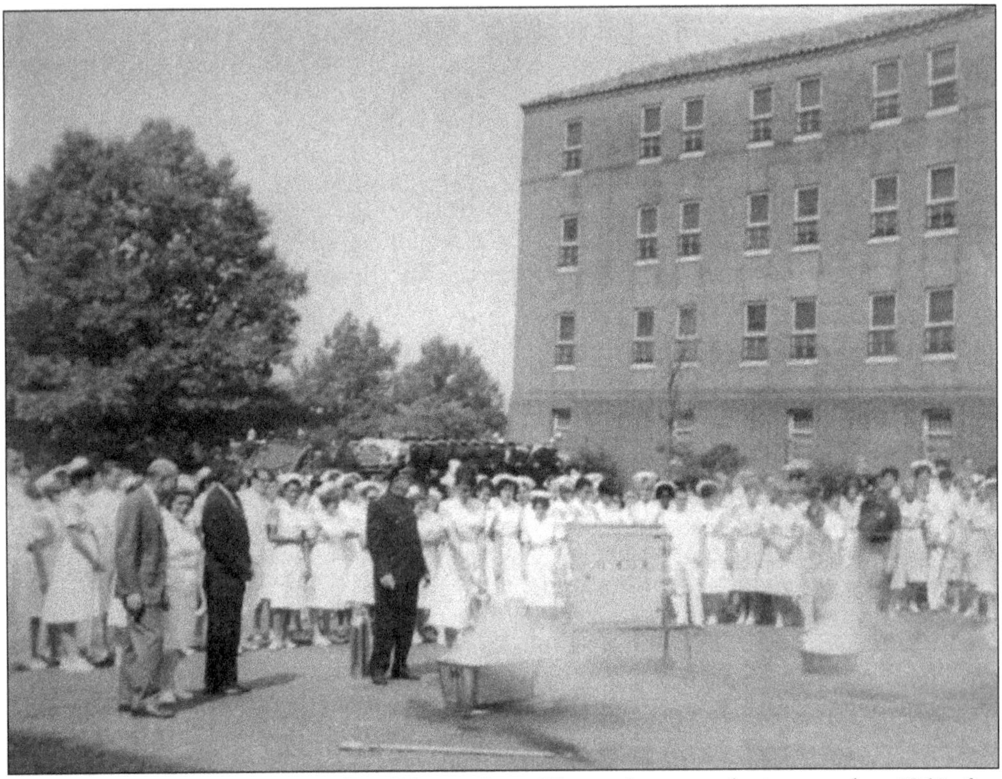

A fire expo for the nursing staff at Pilgrim State Hospital is seen during another 1960s fire prevention day. The cabinet at center reads "Fire Hose," and serves as a prop identical to the ones in the wards. The purpose of the drill was to educate staff on how to operate the hoses during a fire emergency.

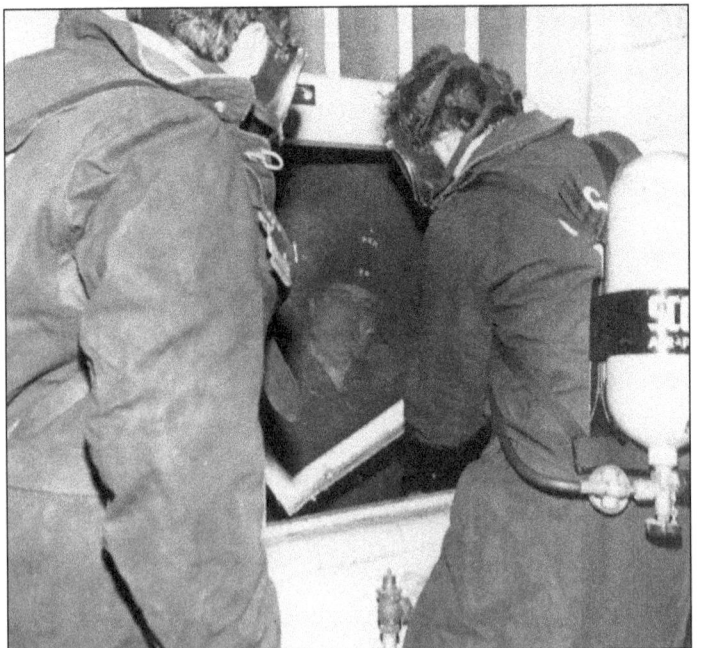

Just as training for the staff at the facilities was important, training drills for the fire service personnel were critical as well. Here, men practice a window-escape drill, where firemen would climb out in full turnout gear with their Scott-brand self-contained breathing apparatus, or SCBA. The SCBA allows for entering and working in conditions that otherwise might not be possible.

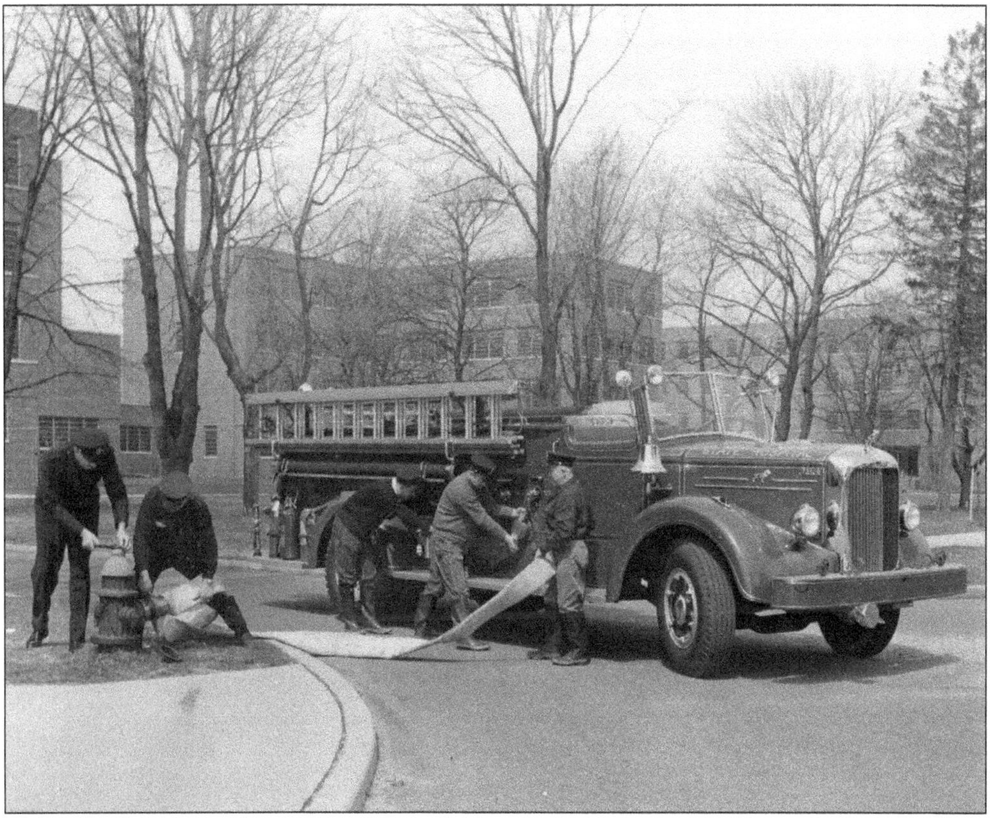

Perhaps one of the most vital tasks for any arriving fire engine is establishing a positive water source. In this 1960s photograph at Central Islip State Hospital, members of the safety department can be seen "hitting a hydrant," or connecting the pumper truck to the fire hydrant. In the background are Buildings 127 and 128.

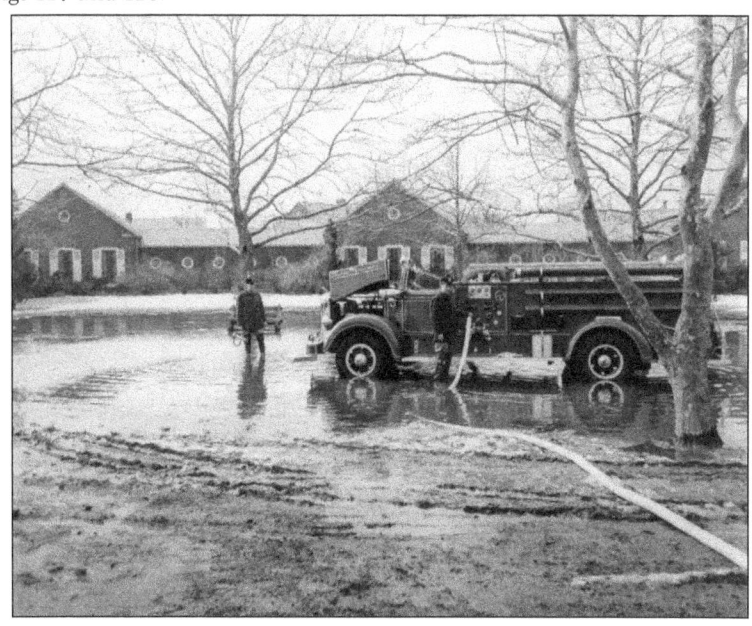

In another photograph at Central Islip State Hospital, a fire engine can be seen operating in winter. A fireman stands in his rubber boots in a large puddle outside of the "Sunburst Building," named for its shape resembling the rays of the rising sun when viewed from above.

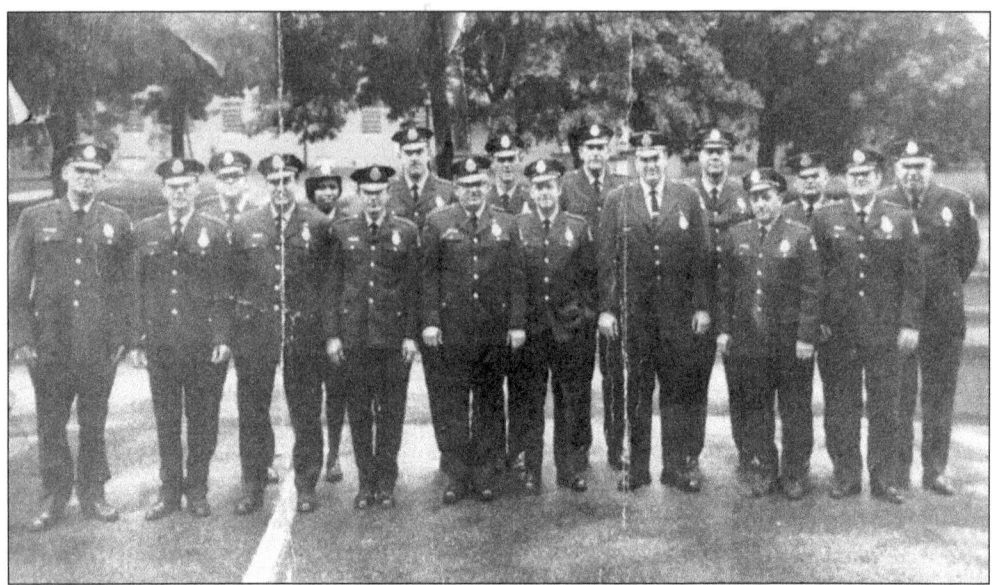

Members of the safety department at Central Islip can be seen in front of the newly constructed Corcoran Complex in the late 1950s. Corcoran, also known as Buildings 127 and 128, was named for Dr. Corcoran, a superintendent of the hospital. The members here are wearing their full-dress coat and uniform shirt.

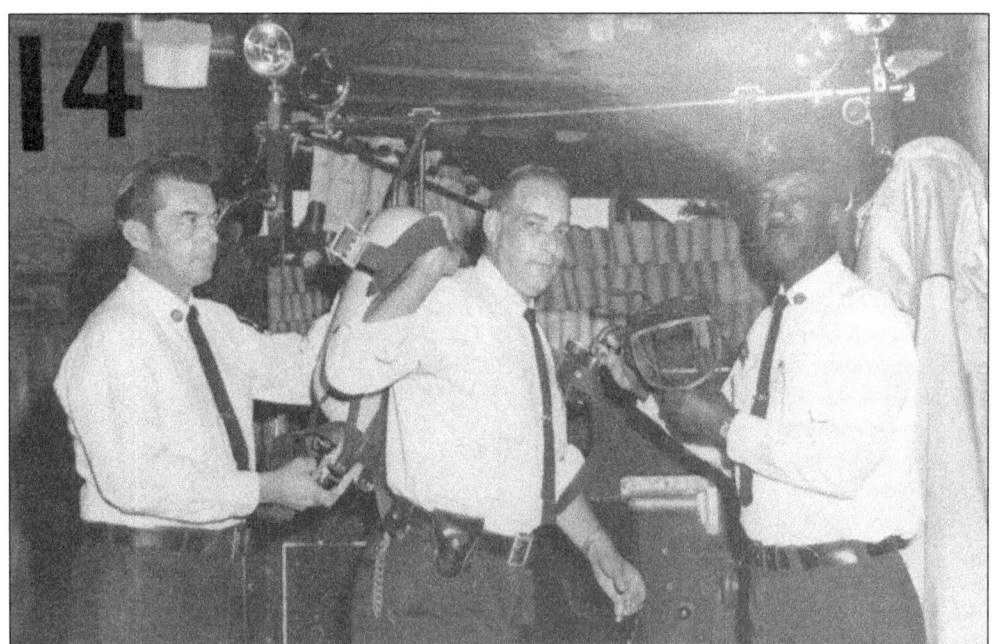

In the 1960s, men at the Pilgrim State Hospital Safety Department can be seen changing out the tank on a SCBA. From left to right are officers Roy Dujat, Harry Sollas, and Teddy Bunce. In the background, a neatly packed fire engine carries an "accordion lay" of hose for firefighting.

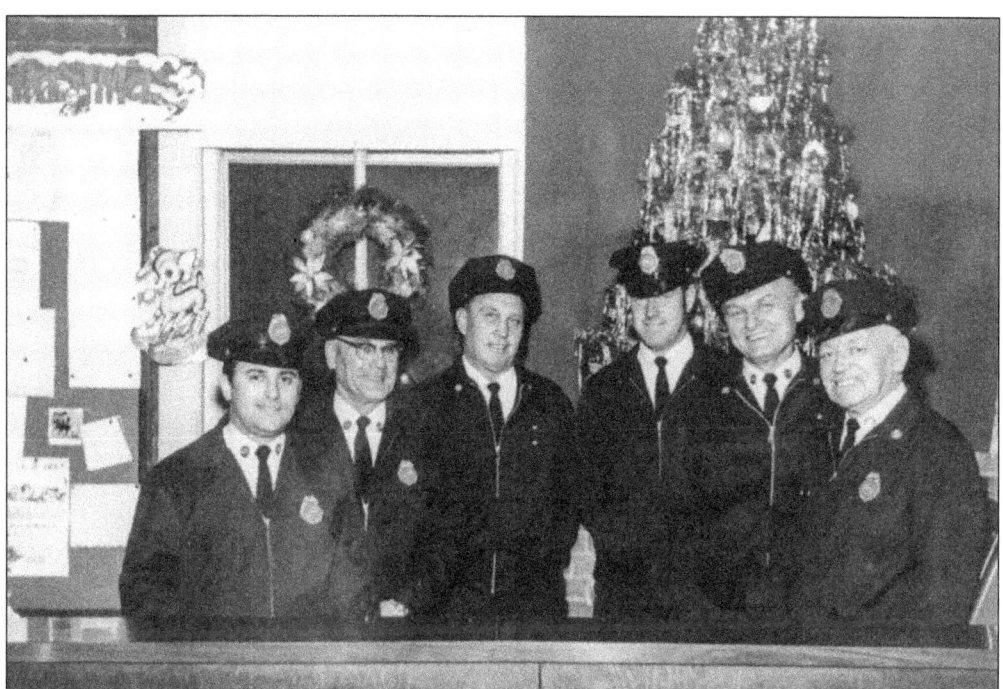

This smiling group of men consists of a few members of the safety department at Kings Park State Hospital near Christmas time. Like many of the nursing staff of the hospitals, safety officers also were required to work 24 hours per day, seven days per week. This would have been one of the first sights for fellow officers or the public who walked into the office area of the safety department building.

As the job of the safety department slowly shifted from fire to law enforcement, the New York State Police initially provided some basic training for safety officers. In this photograph, taken at the assembly hall at Pilgrim State Hospital, Chief Maurice Barry (second from left), Chief Herman Lindeman (second from right), and Chief Julis Cibelli (third from right) can be seen at a ceremony in the 1970s.

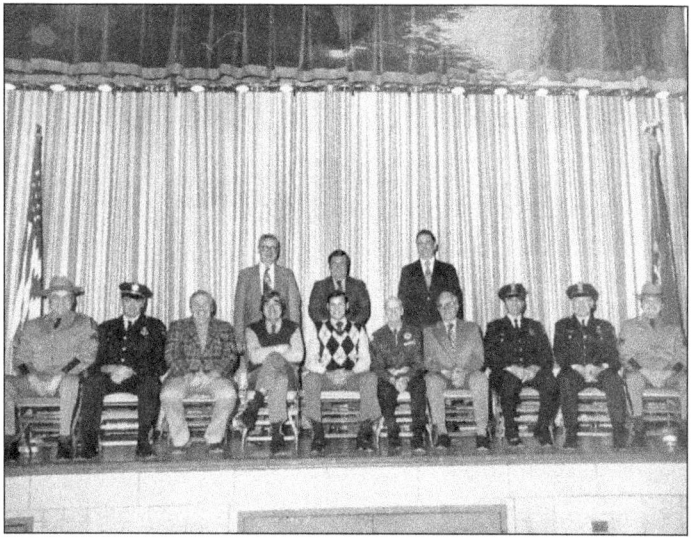

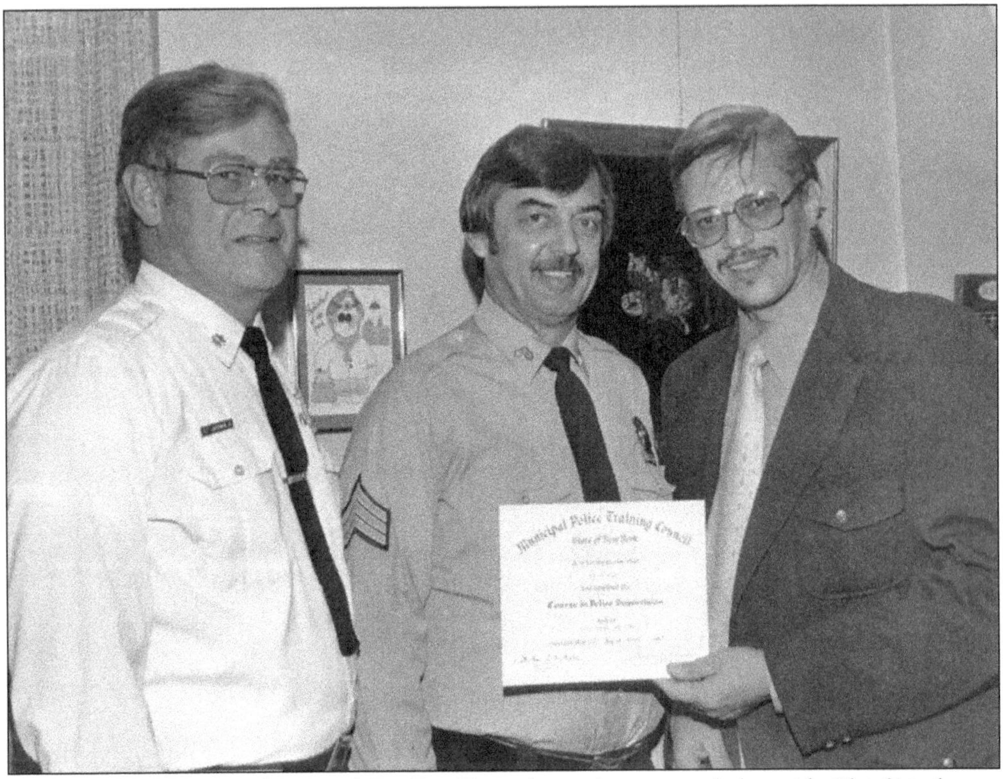

At Pilgrim State Hospital, a proud Sgt. Roy Dujat (center) is pictured alongside Chief Lindeman (left) and hospital director Dr. Iafrate, celebrating his successful completion of a Municipal Police Training Council course in police supervision. In the early days of the facilities, each hospital safety bureau trained to its own standards. As years went on, standards for training were developed at a broader level to include the entire agency.

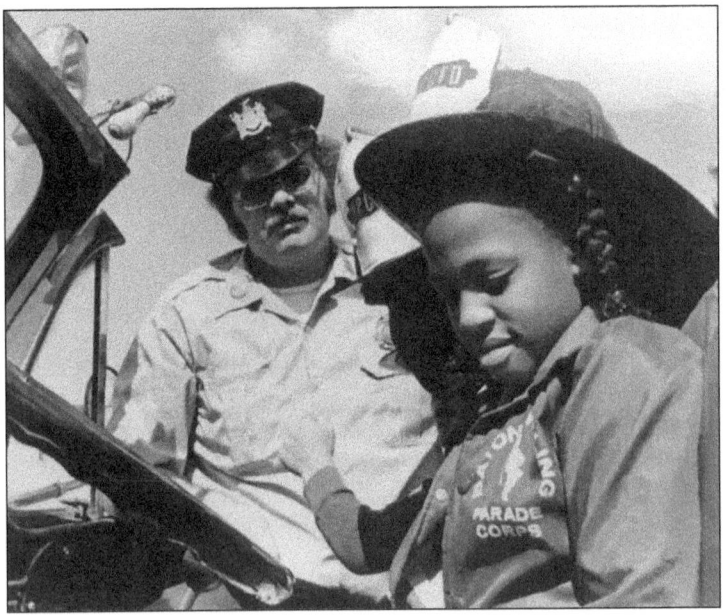

Just like most children, a chance to sit in the neighborhood fire truck was an attractive opportunity for the staff's children at the daycare on the grounds of Pilgrim State Hospital. In the 1970s, safety officer William Cook shows children in fire helmets around the hospital fire engine.

The most distinguishable piece of equipment besides fire engines at the hospital were the patrol cars for the safety department. In this 1970s image, a typical patrol car is seen out on the grounds. The cars carried several different paint schemes over the years. Today, they are solid white with blue lettering.

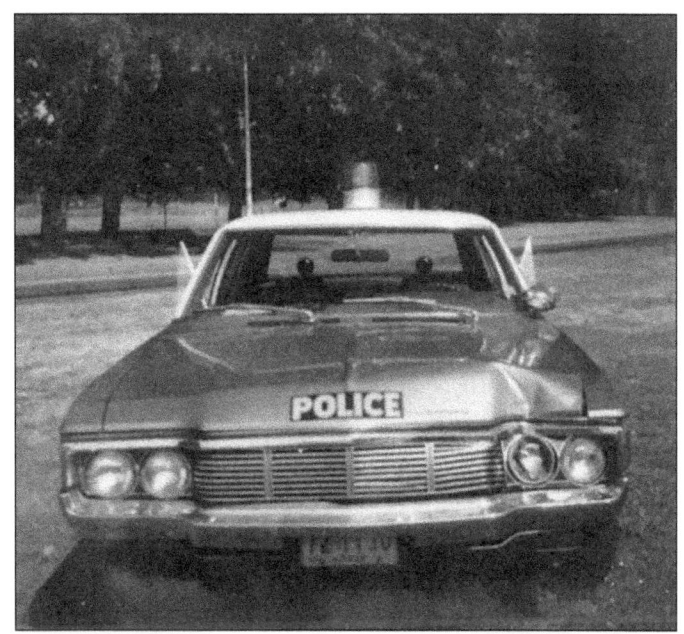

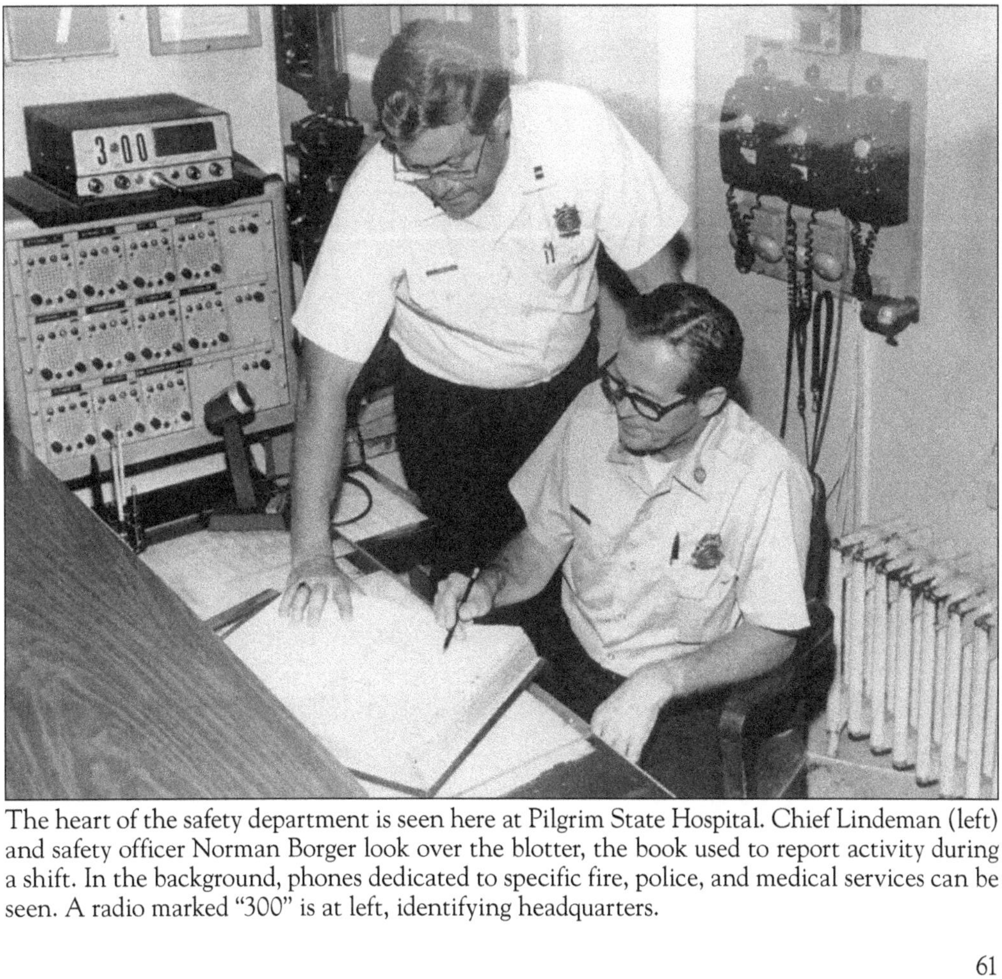

The heart of the safety department is seen here at Pilgrim State Hospital. Chief Lindeman (left) and safety officer Norman Borger look over the blotter, the book used to report activity during a shift. In the background, phones dedicated to specific fire, police, and medical services can be seen. A radio marked "300" is at left, identifying headquarters.

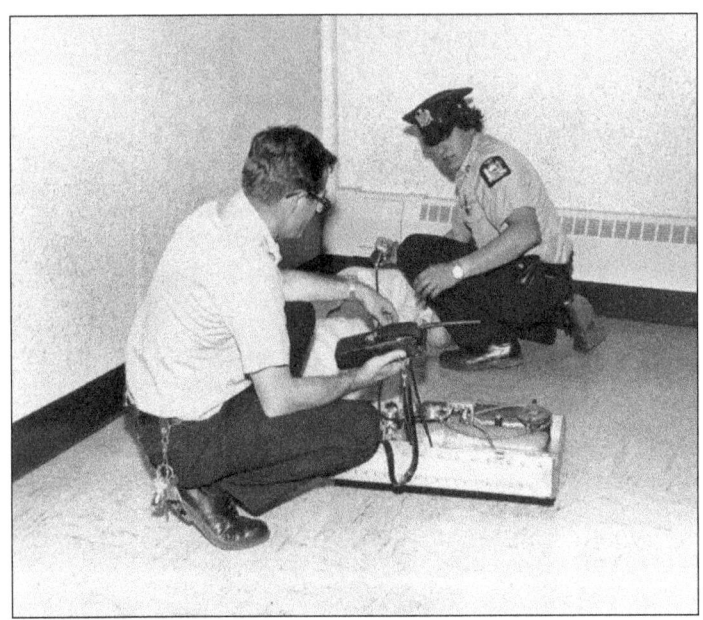

Safety officers are participating in a mass casualty disaster drill at Pilgrim State Hospital. Two officers work together to operate a portable oxygen mask on a mock victim. One tends to the victim as the other relays information to get the appropriate medical intervention.

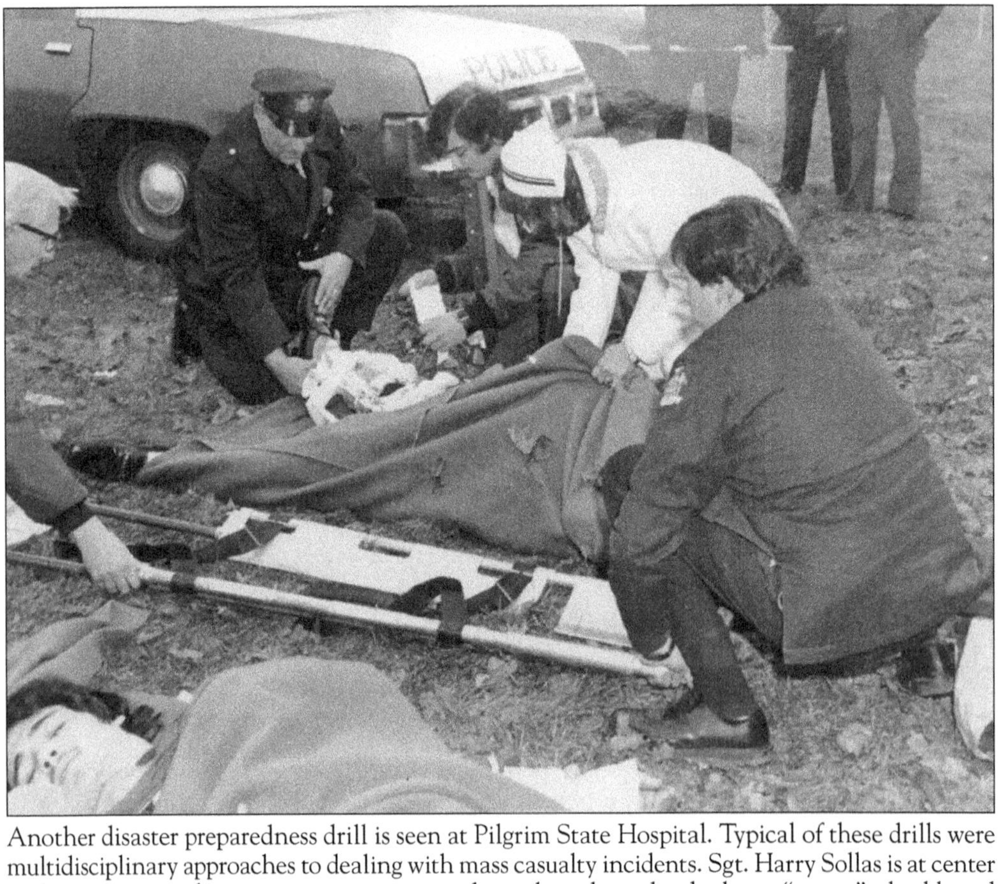

Another disaster preparedness drill is seen at Pilgrim State Hospital. Typical of these drills were multidisciplinary approaches to dealing with mass casualty incidents. Sgt. Harry Sollas is at center with a nurse attending to a victim getting ready to place the individual on a "scoop," a backboard that can hinge open and place a victim on a stretcher easily.

In this 1988 parade photograph, members of the safety department at Pilgrim Psychiatric Center can be seen marching. From left to right are officers Jayne Verticho, Sandy Morrongiello, Angel Colon, and Tommy Bongidrno. In the background, the 80s group buildings were still in operation as Long Island Correctional Facility, a state-run jail that existed briefly on the property.

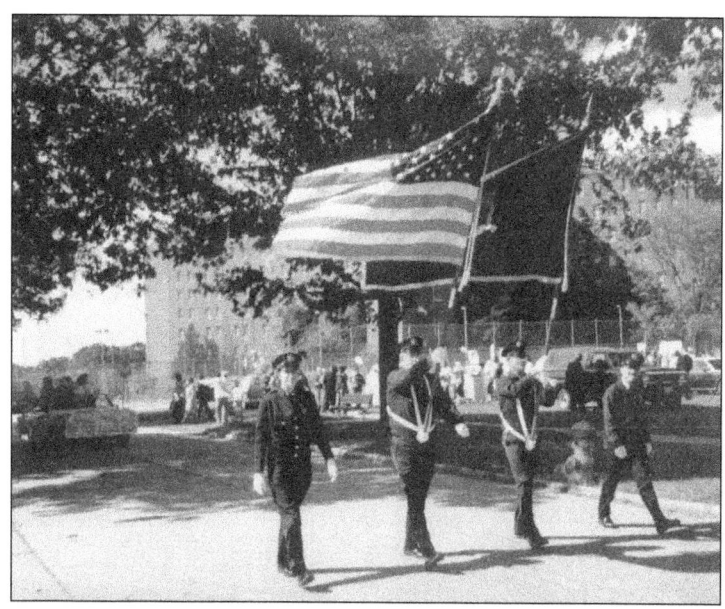

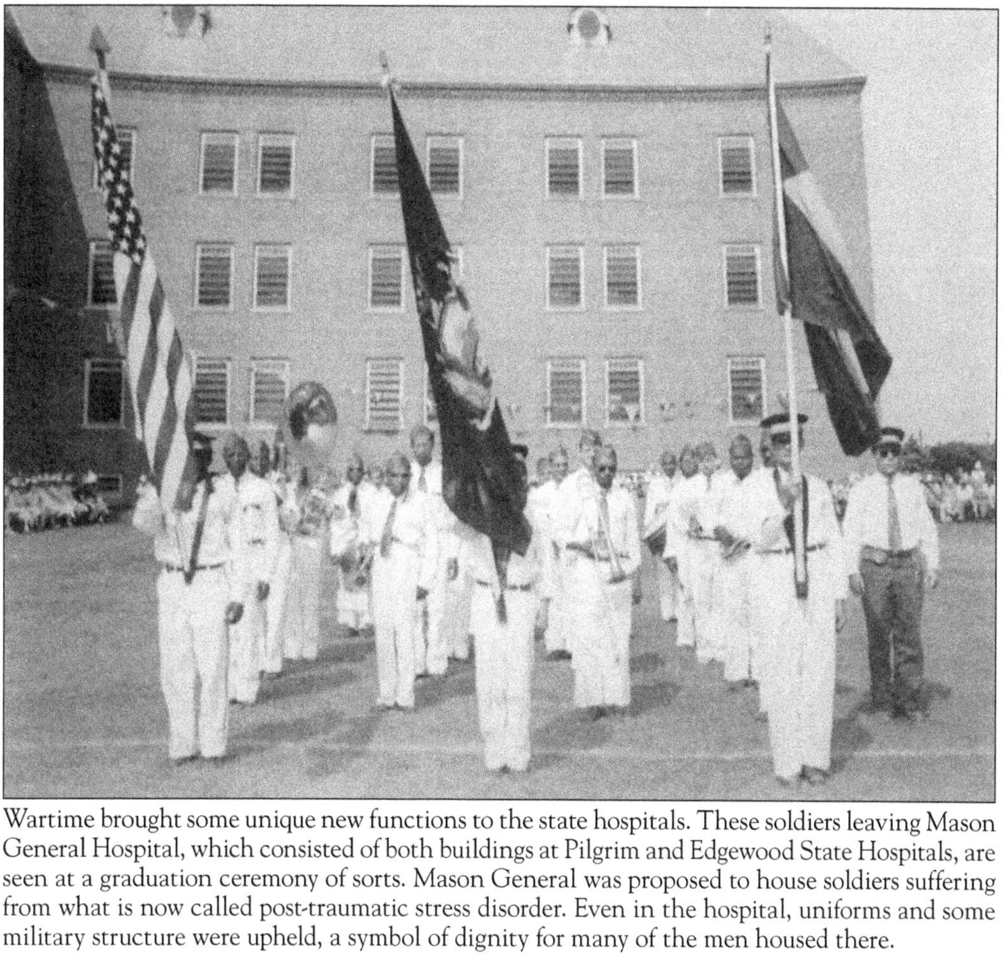

Wartime brought some unique new functions to the state hospitals. These soldiers leaving Mason General Hospital, which consisted of both buildings at Pilgrim and Edgewood State Hospitals, are seen at a graduation ceremony of sorts. Mason General was proposed to house soldiers suffering from what is now called post-traumatic stress disorder. Even in the hospital, uniforms and some military structure were upheld, a symbol of dignity for many of the men housed there.

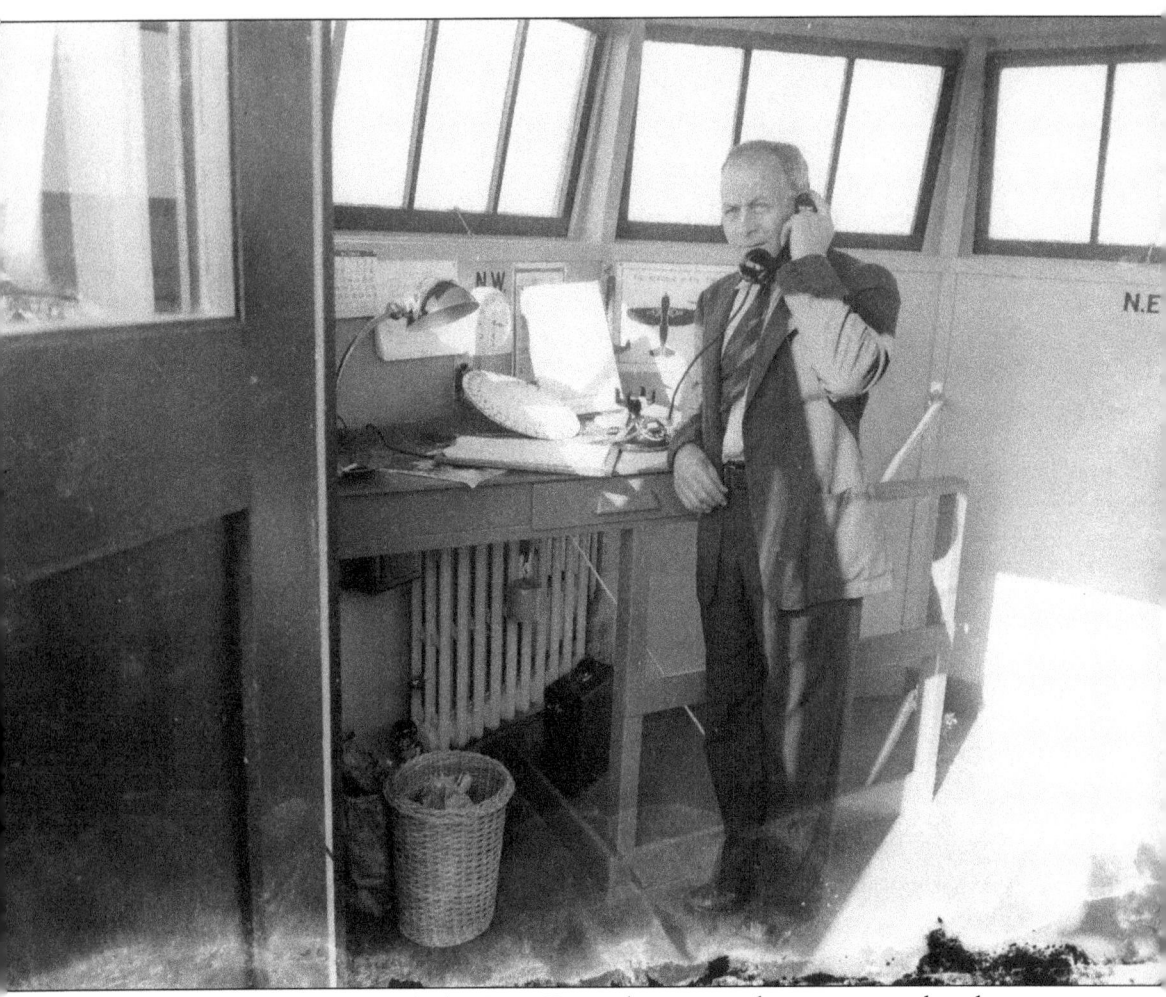

A unique feature of Central Islip State Hospital was a watch station atop the administration building. This observation area was built to spot enemy planes during World War II. On the wall is a drawing of a German aircraft. The letters "N.E" and "N.W." indicated northeast and northwest, for help in reporting the positions of aircraft. An attack on the mainland United States was considered plausible enough for the US War Department to fund the construction of many of these observation stations. In the years following World War II, the station was dismantled.

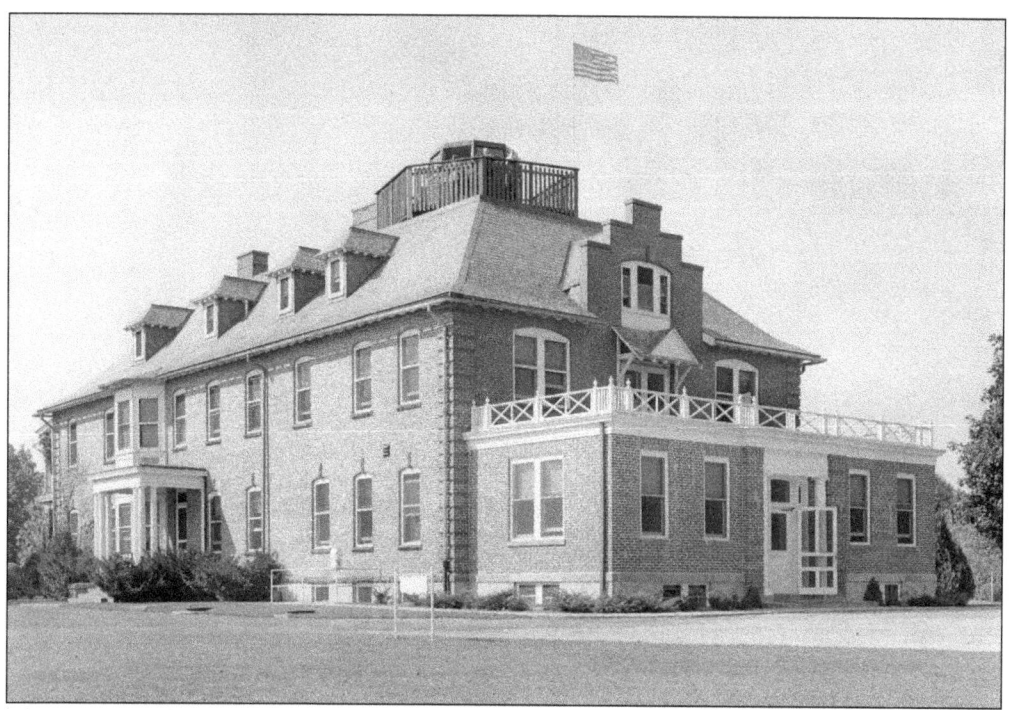

This is a ground view of the watch station at Central Islip. The administration building is proudly flying an American flag. The front entrance faces Carleton Avenue, and the building is set back and surrounded by a meticulously manicured lawn. This building sat vacant for many years before being demolished in 2018 to make way for new construction.

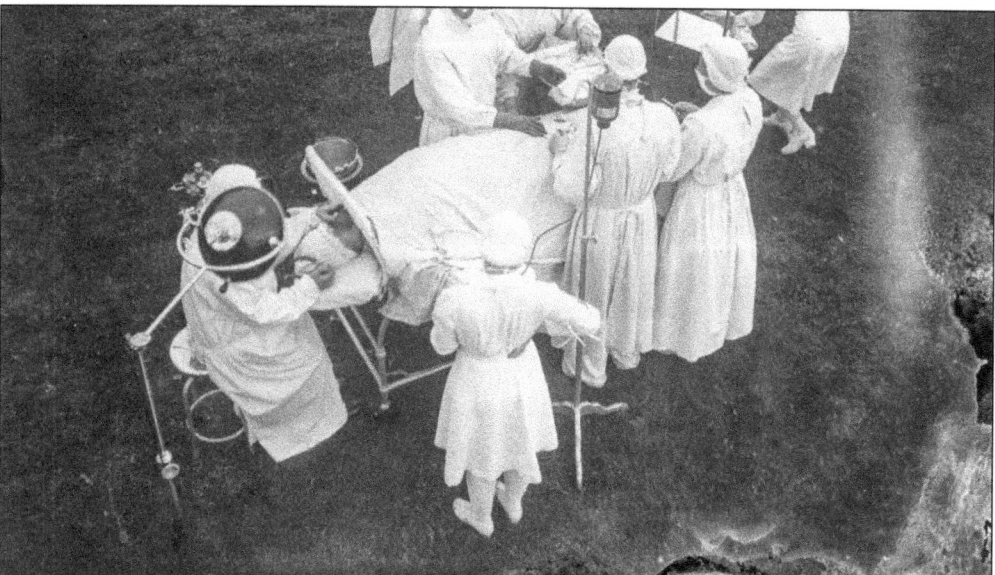

This drill was part of civil defense mass casualty exercises. An outdoor operating center has been set up for a mock surgery. Although primarily a psychiatric hospital, the facility would have been called on for medical assistance in the event of a large-scale incident. Luckily, this type of intervention was never needed during the world wars or any other time that Central Islip State Hospital remained open.

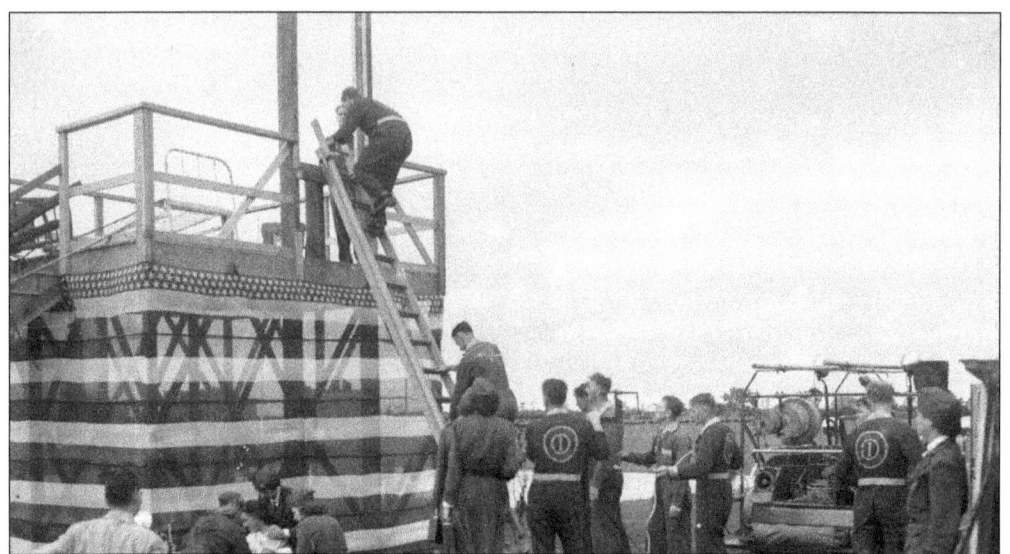

This civil defense drill featured training on window escape and rescue. An elevated wooden platform was constructed at Central Islip State Hospital. On the deck was a simulated hospital room. Although this particular drill was run by civil defense, it was important for staff to be able to evacuate themselves and patients during any emergency.

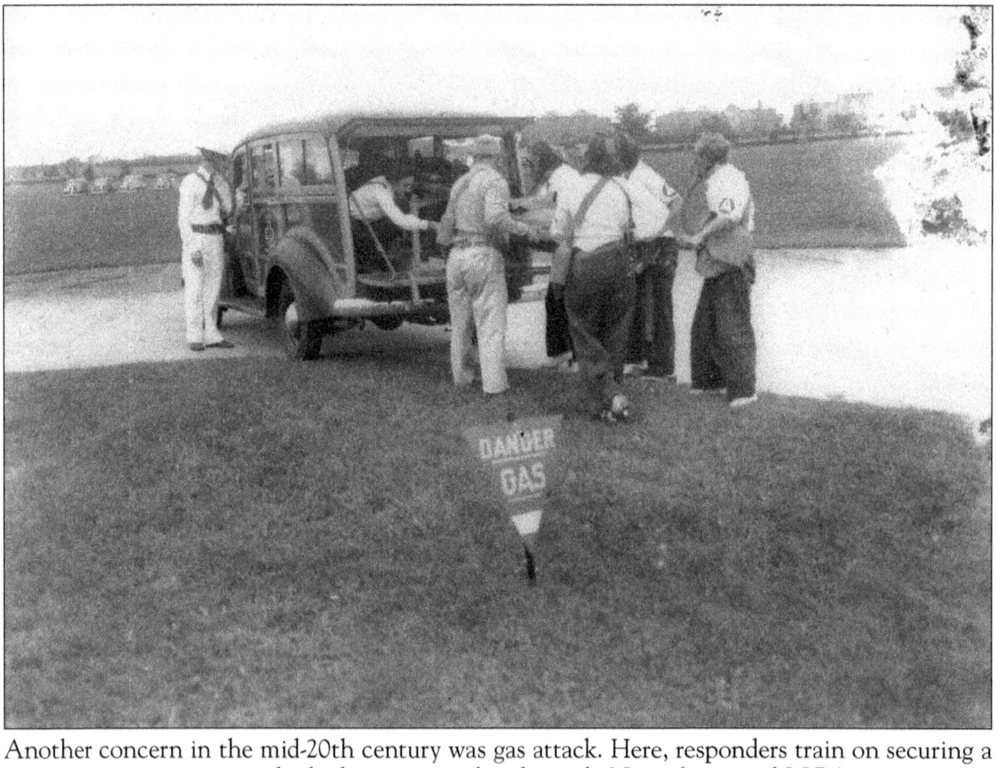

Another concern in the mid-20th century was gas attack. Here, responders train on securing a patient into a transport vehicle during a simulated attack. Note the use of SCBA apparatus. In the distance, staff apartment housing can be seen at Central Islip State Hospital.

Four

THE FARMS AND SHOPS

Farming at the state hospitals served dual functions. Food production to sustain the vast numbers of staff and patients living on the grounds was one, since growing food onsite saved substantial amounts of money. The other function was therapeutic. In the early 20th century, farming work was considered a very effective treatment adjunct for patients. Moral treatment was the principal model at most institutions of the era. Providing occupation that was in turn beneficial to the institution made good sense to most of the managers at such facilities. At Central Islip State Hospital in 1903, the largest percentage of patients who were employed at the hospital were farm and garden workers. This seemed to be effective for many patients, as it had the benefit of time spent outdoors in a relaxed setting and allowed for a lenient learning curve. Paid farmers were onsite and were responsible for the commercial raising of crops and livestock. Superintendent Smith at Central Islip remarked, "We must not forget to mention patients' individual farms and gardens which were growing in number and size every year and the quality and quantity of vegetables produced are better as they become more proficient in the art of farming."

Produce from Central Islip was routinely exhibited at the Suffolk County Fair and American Institution Fair in New York City, receiving awards as well as honorable mentions. By 1940, approximately 335 acres were used for farmland. A total of 118 cows were on hand, in addition to 330 pigs. Up to 500 patients daily were engaged in activities on the grounds. Similarly, Pilgrim State Hospital, upon its commissioning, had 800 acres of farmland. Another monumental support function on the grounds were the various tradesmen working at the hospitals' shops. Almost all necessary parts, repairs, laundry, and moderate renovation projects were done in house for many decades. Patient workers frequently aided in these areas and often gained technical knowledge leading to jobs upon discharge.

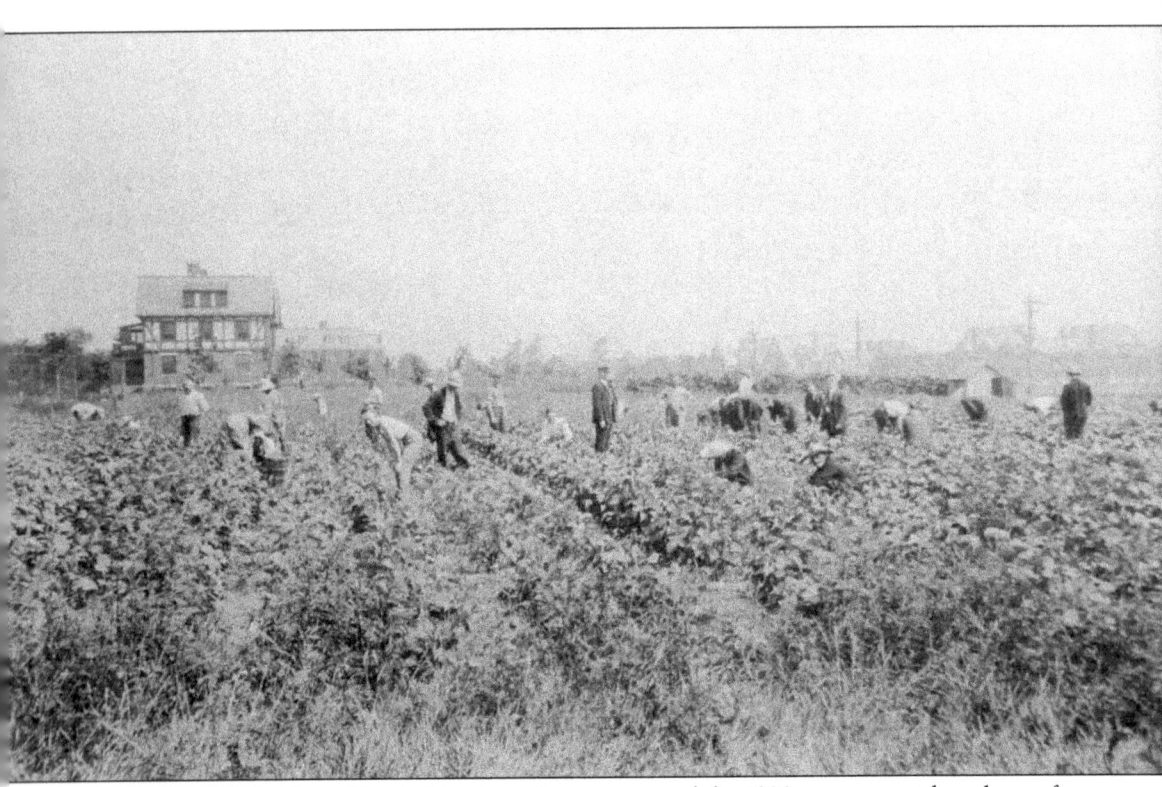

At Central Islip State Hospital in the springtime around the 1920s, men are picking beans for use in the hospital kitchens. The workers are wearing straw hats, likely made at the facility, to provide some shade. At center, wearing a suit and hat, an officer of the hospital, a ranking member of the administration, is evaluating conditions. In the background, the gable roofs of the dining hall and ward buildings in the Smith Group are visible. This plot was one of several farming areas on the grounds. Beans grew well and often to excess in the sandy, well-drained soil of Long Island. Excess produce was canned for use in the colder months or sold at market.

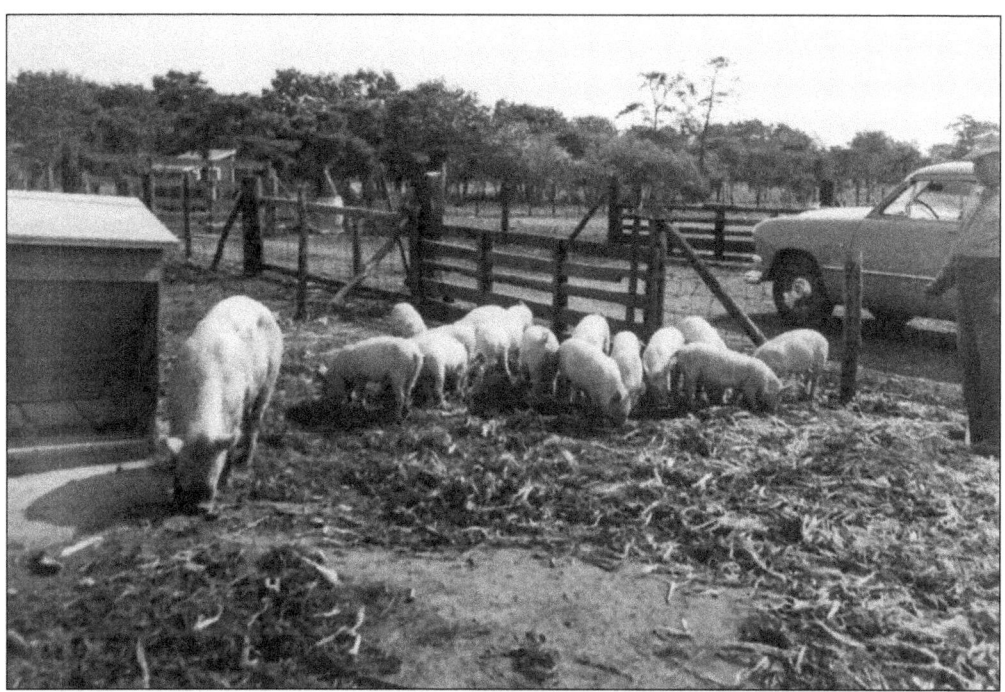

Aside from large quantities of produce, livestock was raised and processed in sizable numbers at the state hospitals. Pigs in particular were easily to sustain because they could be fed leftover scraps from the dining halls. This allowed for an inexpensive supplement to augment traditional pig feed, and less waste of food products. In these photographs taken in the 1960s at Pilgrim State Hospital, pigs are shown at the hospital farm. In the distance, several other droves, or groups of young pigs, can be seen alongside their mothers. Men working on the farm stand in the background on a spring day.

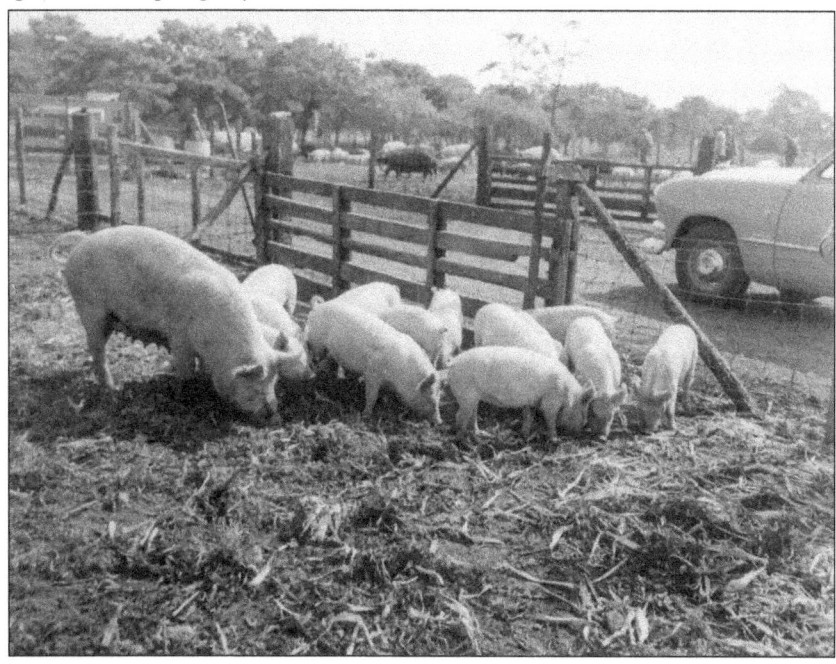

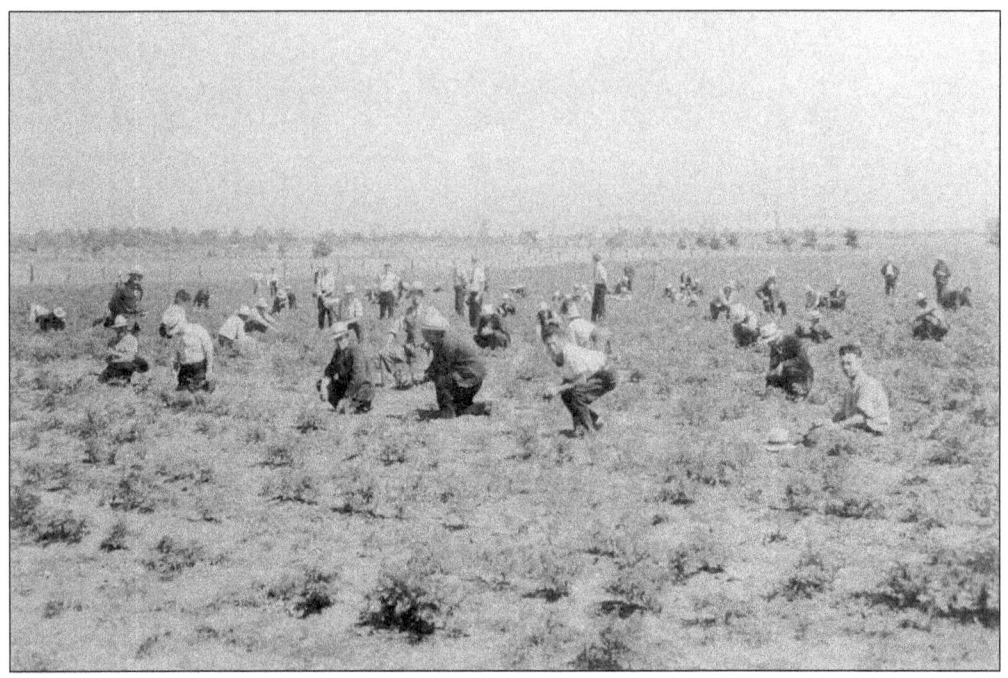

One of the most performed and necessary tasks on the farms was weeding. Usually, this was accomplished in squads of multiple people. Above, men can be seen weeding the farm area facing what is now Carleton Avenue at Central Islip State Hospital. Below, men weed the field adjacent to the administration building, which can be seen at left. Weeding was a task that individuals with limited experience could jump into and successfully complete with little direction. Facilitating success in the tasks patients performed was the goal of the staff, providing them a feeling of pride and accomplishment that could be used to build up other areas of their lives.

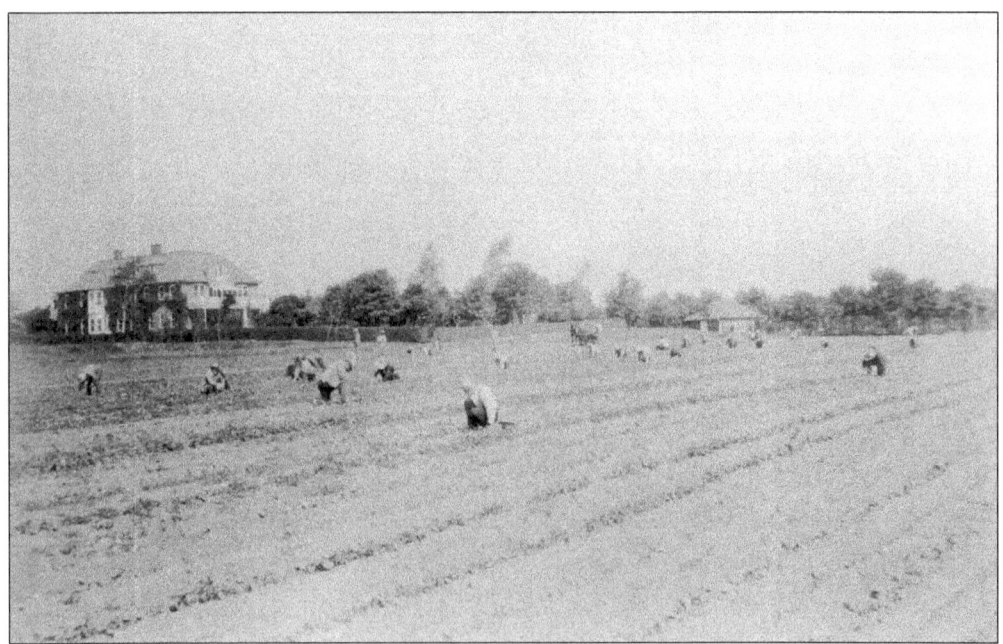

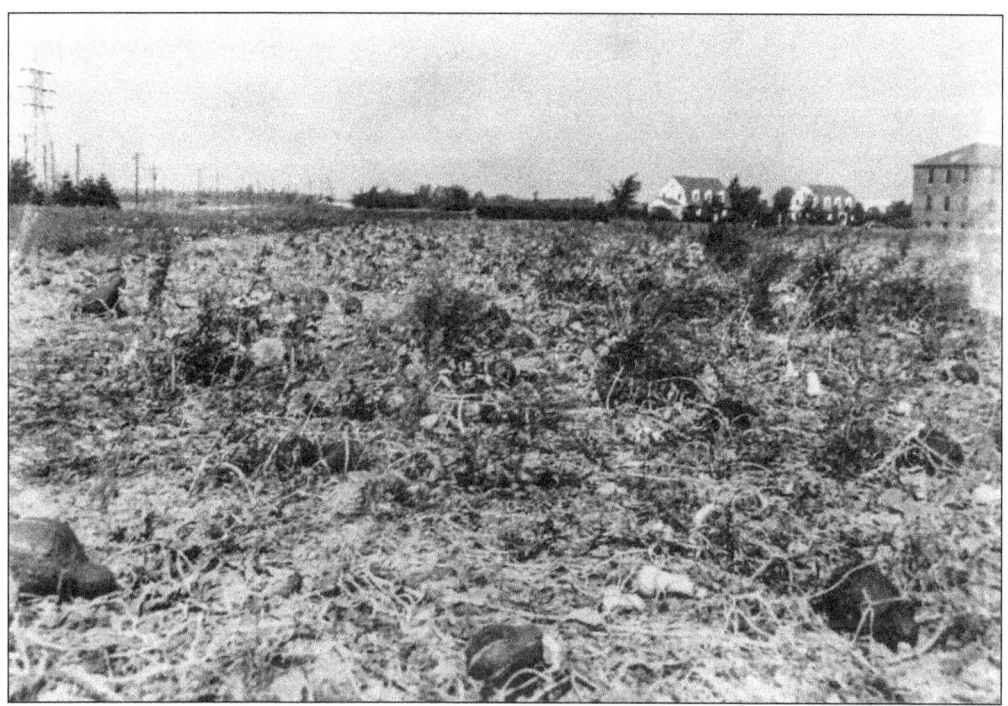

The same area of farmland is shown at two different times. Above, the fall harvest of gourds and squash can be seen in a seemingly boundless farm field at Pilgrim State Hospital. Below, in later years, the same patch of land can be seen unsown. As decades went on, the once-thriving farms at the state hospitals diminished and were eventually shuttered in the early 1970s. This parcel of land was sold off and converted into a park, as was Suffolk Community College, in an 800-acre deal. The buildings in the background can be found today in use at the county college along Crooked Hill Road.

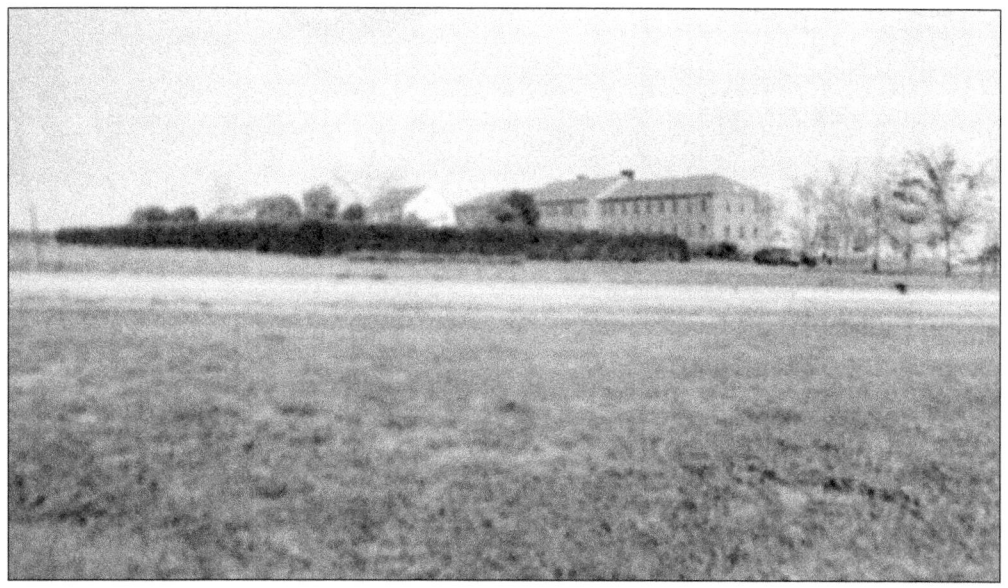

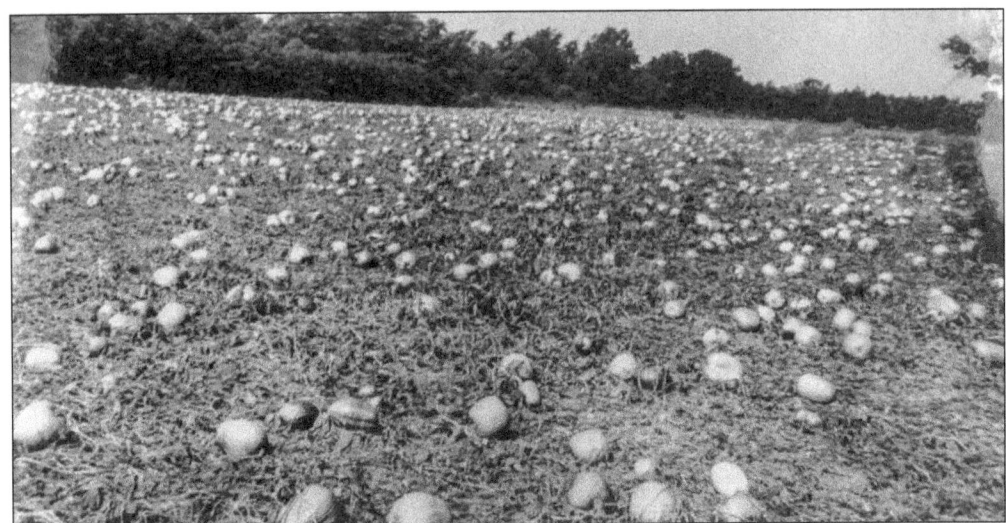

A regular sight at Pilgrim State Hospital in the heyday of farm operations, a field of pumpkins sits ready for harvest. This fall crop provided more than the fillings for pies to be baked in the hospital kitchen. Pumpkin carving provided a recreational activity for patients all around the hospital. Fall dance socials would be adorned with pumpkins, corn stalks, and gourds, all grown at the facility farm.

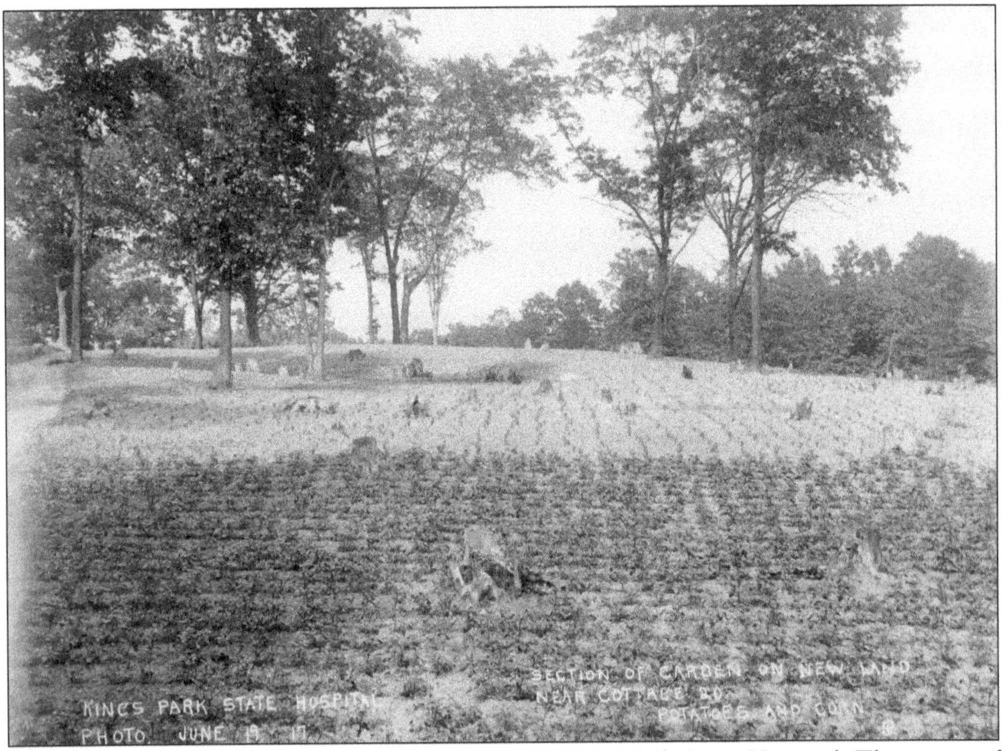

Corn and potatoes were two important staples at Kings Park State Hospital. Their ease of growth and abundant yields made them ideal for feeding hundreds of people. In this spring 1917 photograph, a newly cleared and planted section of land is used to grow corn and potato crops.

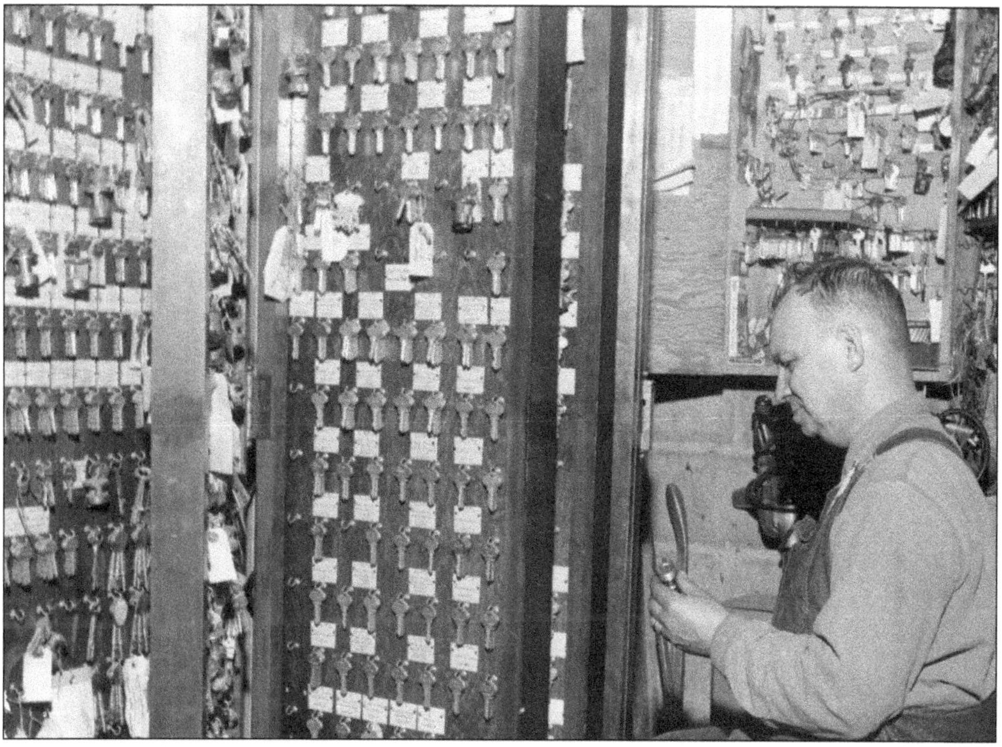

Thousands of doors, cabinets, windows, and other items were required to work 365 days a year. As building uses changed, so too would its locks, in order to maintain security. In the early days, skeleton keys were returned to a supervisor at the completion of duty. As a result of increasingly modern locksmithing, complex key systems were developed to ensure that different levels of staff had access to the areas appropriate to their job. Above, the Central Islip State Hospital locksmith shop can be seen. Below, Pilgrim State Hospital's locksmith shop is shown sometime in the 1960s.

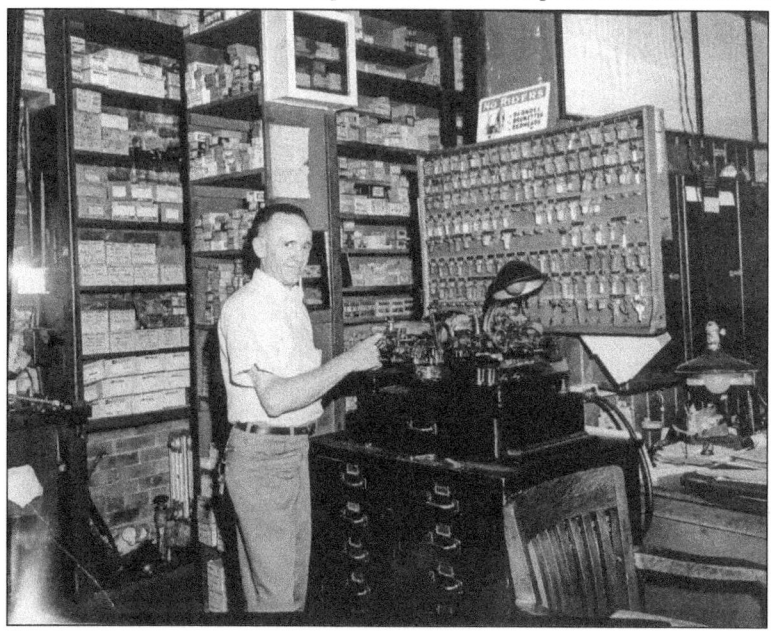

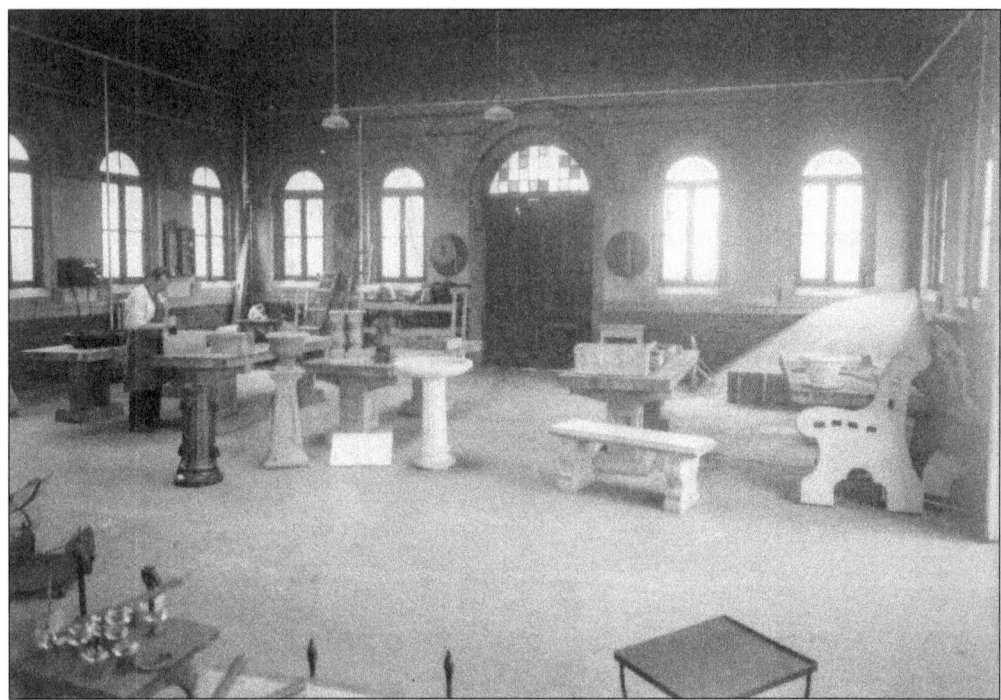

Innumerable quantities of fixtures at Kings Park State Hospital were constructed of concrete for durability and ease of maintenance. Outdoor benches, birdbaths, and flower boxes like the ones pictured above were produced in the cement shop at Kings Park. The cement shops did not just make ornamental items; construction materials were also produced. Below, men mix cement (left) to be placed in a form (right). The end result would be blocks suitable for construction or repair on the hospital grounds at Central Islip State Hospital. At left is a stack of completed blocks.

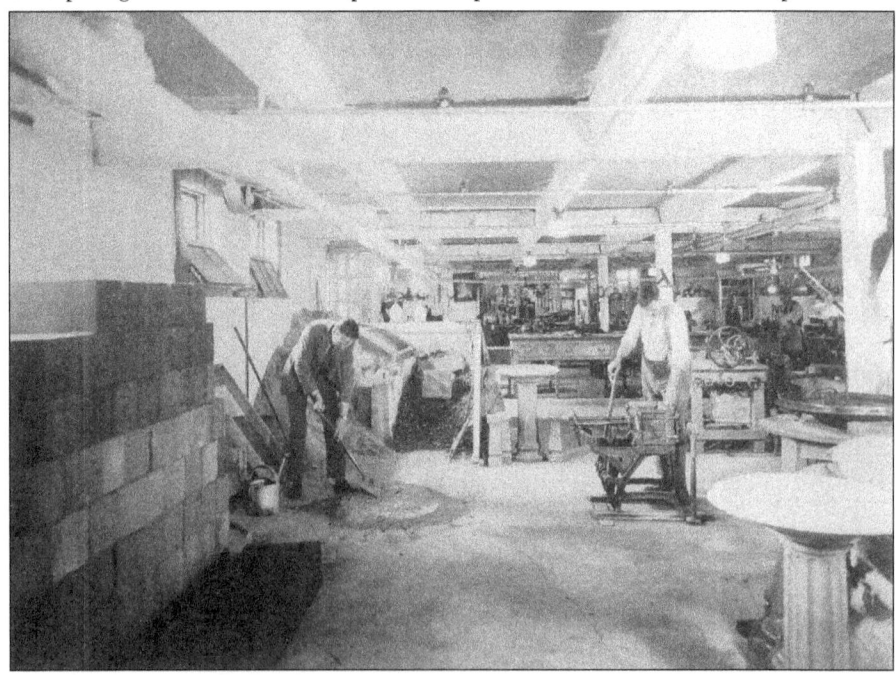

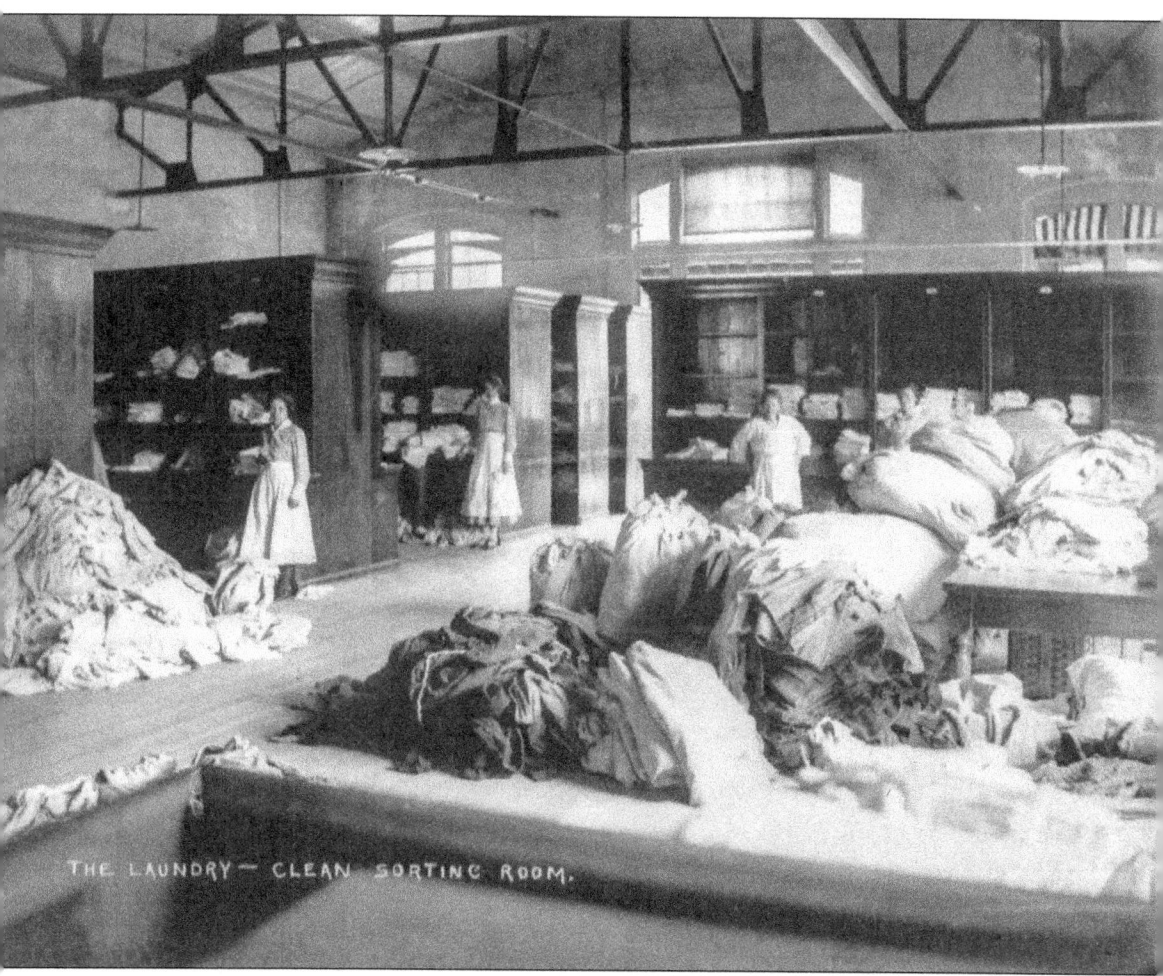

Laundry service was vital to daily operations at the hospitals. Thousands of staff and patients relied on a systematic approach to collecting, cleaning, and distributing articles of clothing in order for a speedy return. Large canvas bags were marked with the building and ward for soiled linens to be placed in, and securely closed with large safety pins. Full bags were transported to the laundry, separated, and washed. After washing in large steam-powered machines and drying, laundry was carted out to a clean sorting room, like the one shown here. In the sorting room, linens were arranged by item and size and then placed back into circulation. Clothes would be returned to the unit from which they arrived along with their cleaned laundry bag. Each building had specific times and dates to pick up and drop off laundry. This photograph was taken in Building 5 at Kings Park State Hospital in the 1920s. (Courtesy of the Kings Park Heritage Museum.)

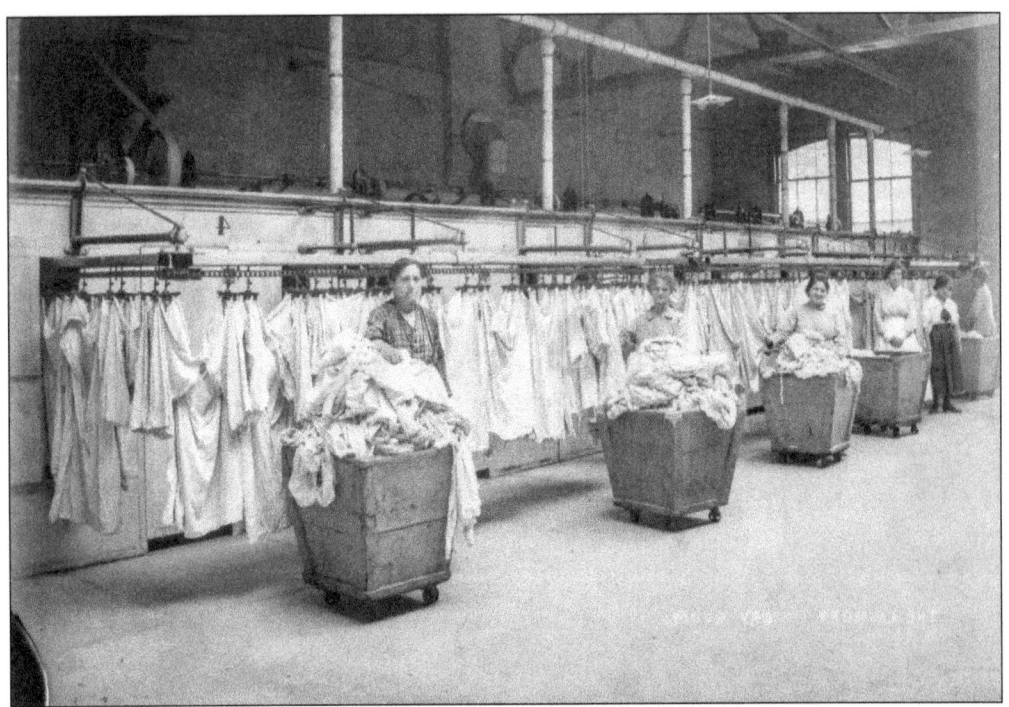

After washing, laundry was hung on mechanized racks for drying. Above, at Kings Park State Hospital, women are hanging up nightgowns for drying around the 1920s. The conveyor-style rack passed the wet clothing through heated blowers to speed the drying time. Below, men work in the laundry press shop. Here, linens and clothes were steam pressed to ensure a tidy appearance. Men and women were not permitted to fraternize during work at the time these photographs were taken. Men working in the laundry often operated the washing machines and presses, and carted clothes around. Women primarily worked in the sorting and sewing areas. (Courtesy of the Kings Park Heritage Museum.)

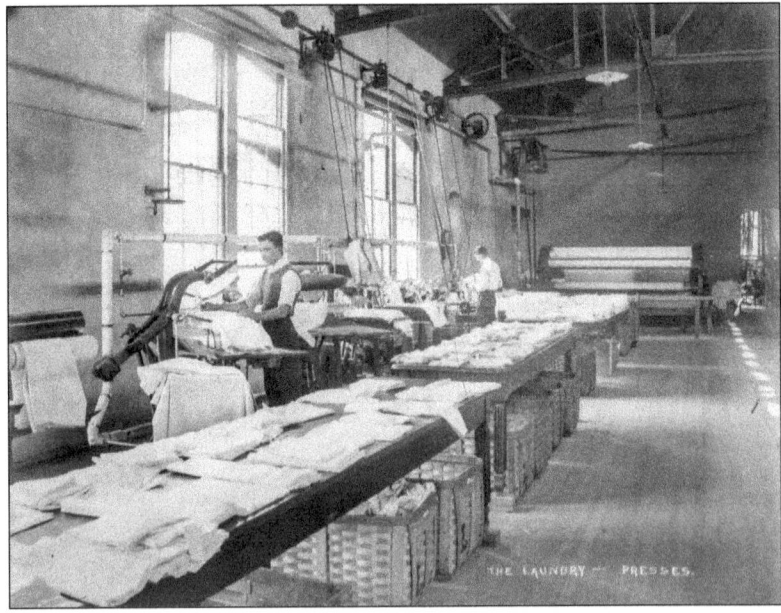

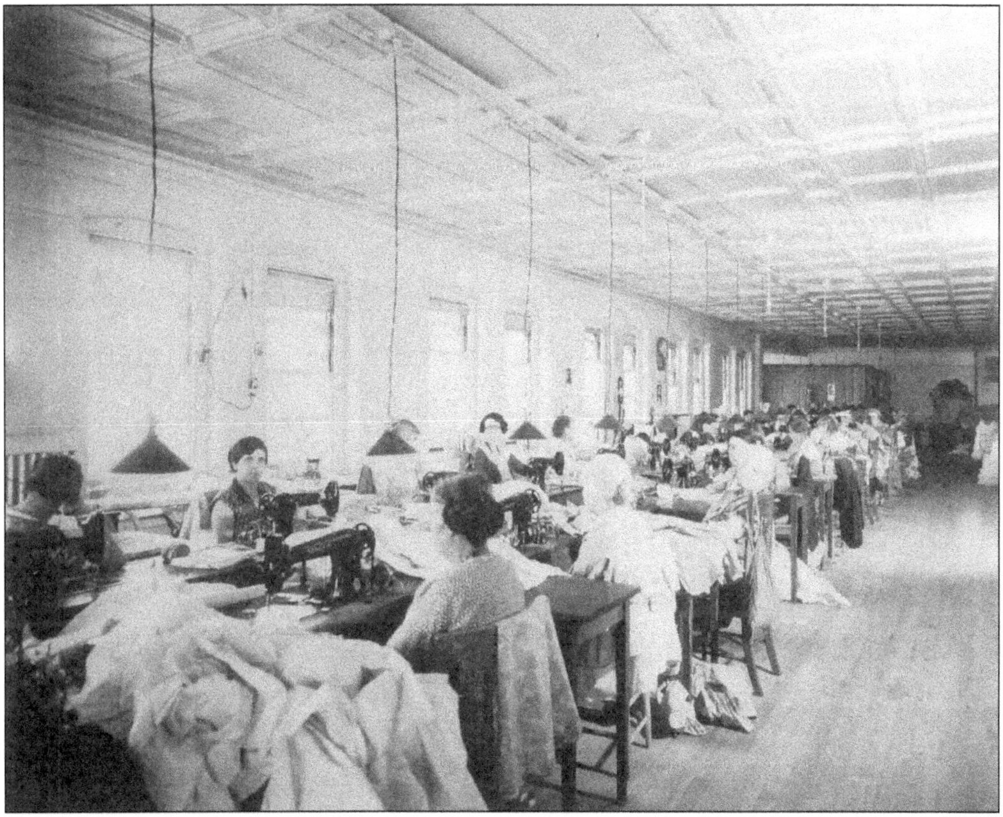

Clothing was both made and repaired at the state hospitals. This kept costs low, and the money saved was used to purchase better materials, providing patients and staff with quality clothing. Here, a sewing room at the South Colony at Central Islip State Hospital is seen in operation.

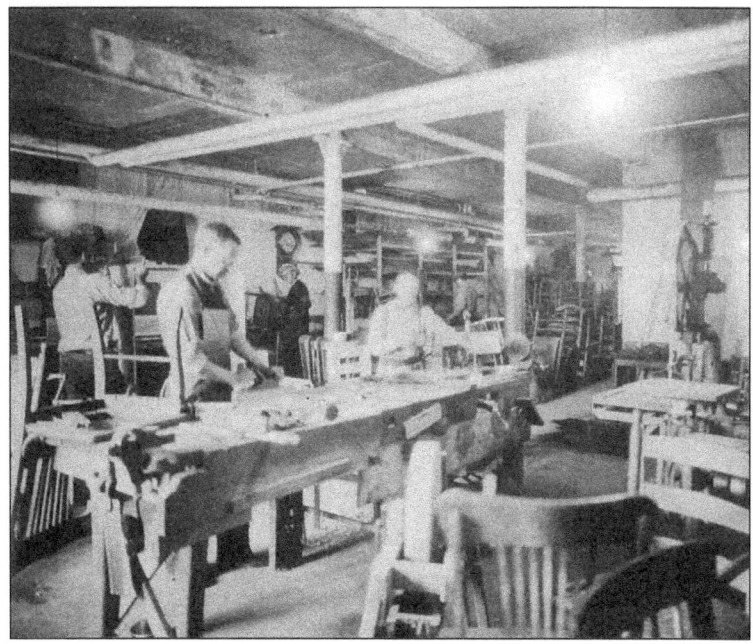

Furniture was also made and repaired on the grounds. In this 1930s image at Central Islip State Hospital, men are working in the chair and cane shop. Many chairs had cane seats and backing that often required repair from wear and tear. In the foreground is a completed chair.

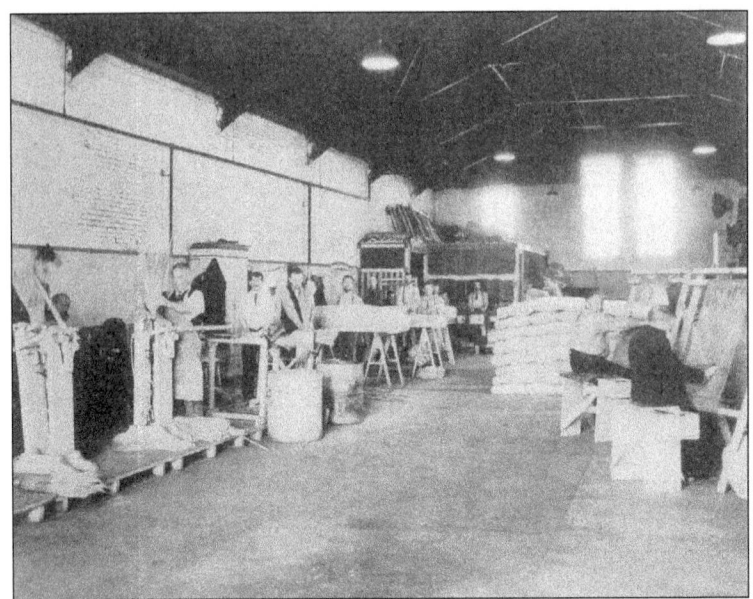

Two seemingly unrelated household items were produced together at Central Islip State Hospital in the early 20th century. This photograph of the broom and mattress shop shows the production process of both. At left, men attach hard bristle ends to broom handles. At right, men weave and stuff the inside of mattresses with straw and cotton.

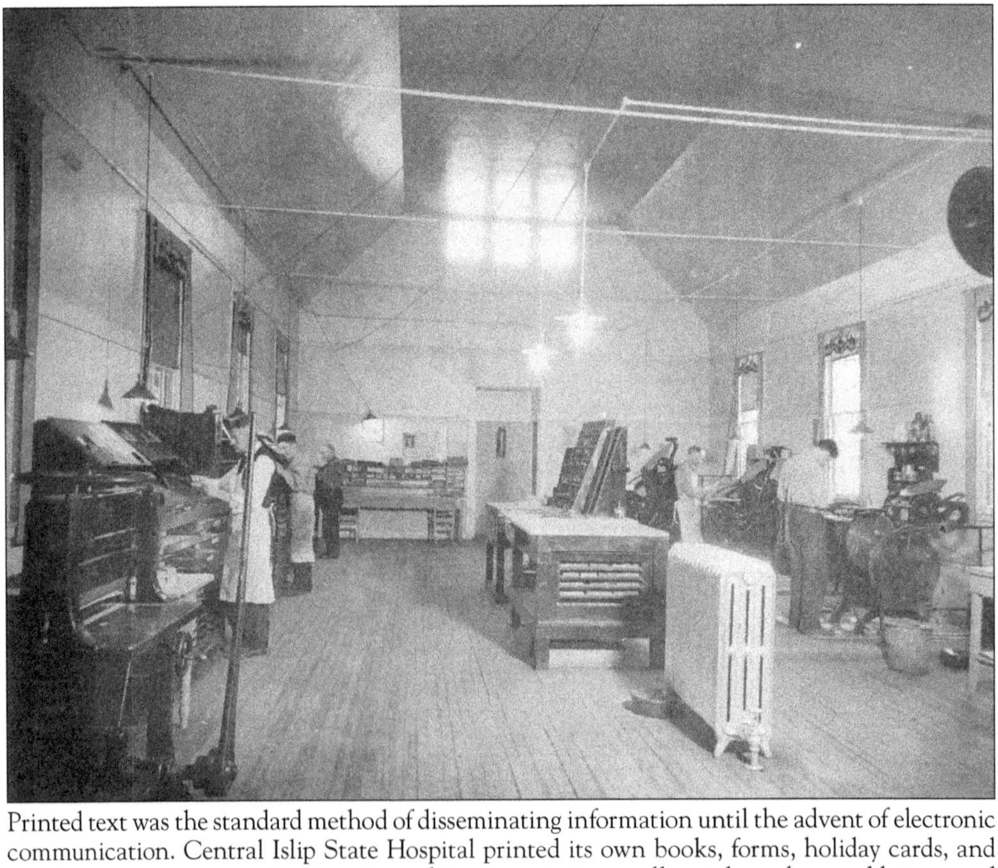

Printed text was the standard method of disseminating information until the advent of electronic communication. Central Islip State Hospital printed its own books, forms, holiday cards, and even its own newspaper. At center is a cabinet containing small metal numbers and letters used to compose text for the printing presses.

Five

LIFE AND ACTIVITIES ON THE GROUNDS

Life at the farm colonies was seldom lacking in work to be performed. Everything from clearing fields to weaving baskets was completed by individuals on the grounds. Patients were encouraged, but never forced, to work in all areas of the facilities except healthcare. This work helped many patients balance routines and define self-worth. Learning a new trade or pursuing an existing one led to successful and wholesome lives for patients after discharge. Comprehensive therapeutic interventions were furnished to individuals. However, work therapy allowed patients unique bonding opportunities with peers and staff. Some trustworthy patients even held certain hospital keys. They were sometimes referred to as "honor patients."

Working in a hospital in the 19th century was more than a job for the employees—it was a way of life. Staff worked with patients in various capacities, lived in adjoining parts of ward buildings, and ate in the same dining halls. Staff was to ensure patients were awoken each day at 6:00 a.m. in order to be in the dining halls and fed. By 7:00 a.m., able-bodied patients went to their respective squads, or work crews, on the grounds. Lunch was at 12:00 p.m. sharp. Patients washed and were to be ready to work again by 1:00 p.m. By 5:00 p.m., all work was over for the day. In the evening and on weekends, patients attended social events, movies, sports, and religious services. Medical clinics and occupational and psychiatric therapy were held in groups during weekdays before 5:00 p.m. Routines provided patients with stability and expectations for days of the week.

Until the late 20th century, moral therapy, the principal psychosocial rehabilitation treatment at the state hospitals, involved an emphasis on work, music, dance, art, and cooperative activity. As a result, the activities department, later known as occupational therapy, provided the greatest amount of group treatment until the 1940s.

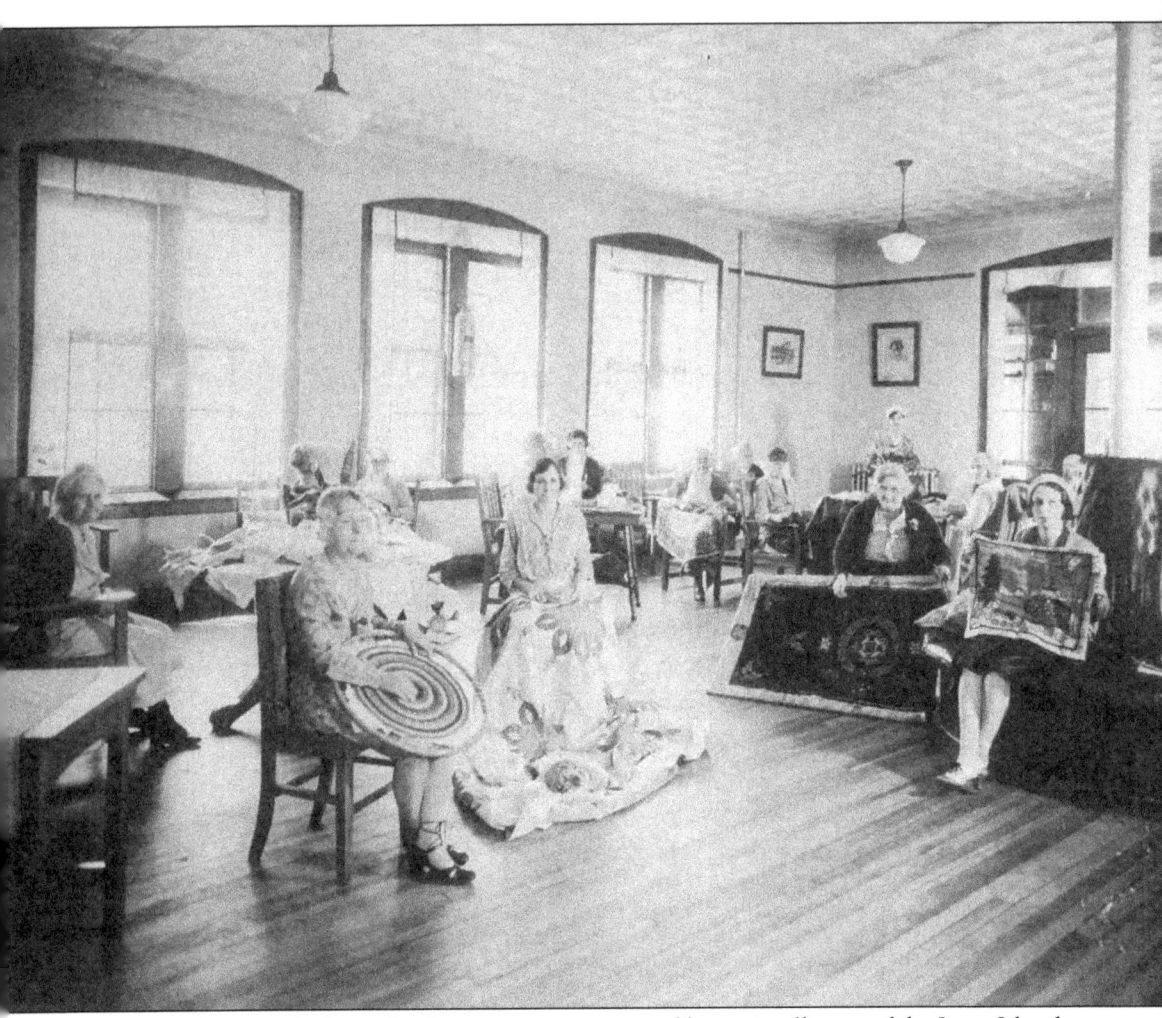

Until the 1970s, both staff and patients were separated by sex in all areas of the Long Island state hospitals. Fraternizing between males and females was prohibited, and only permitted at social events or dances hosted in the assembly halls. Pictured above in a female unit during the 1920s at Central Islip State Hospital, women can be seen in a day room of the Smith Group. Note the ornate, high tin ceiling, quarter-sawn pine flooring, and large arched windows, which allowed much light and airflow. The women were crafting rugs, quilts, and other needlework items. Such items were often placed on display at occupational therapy exhibits or utilized around the hospital. Upon close inspection, the items produced by the women are extremely detailed, displaying a notable level of talent.

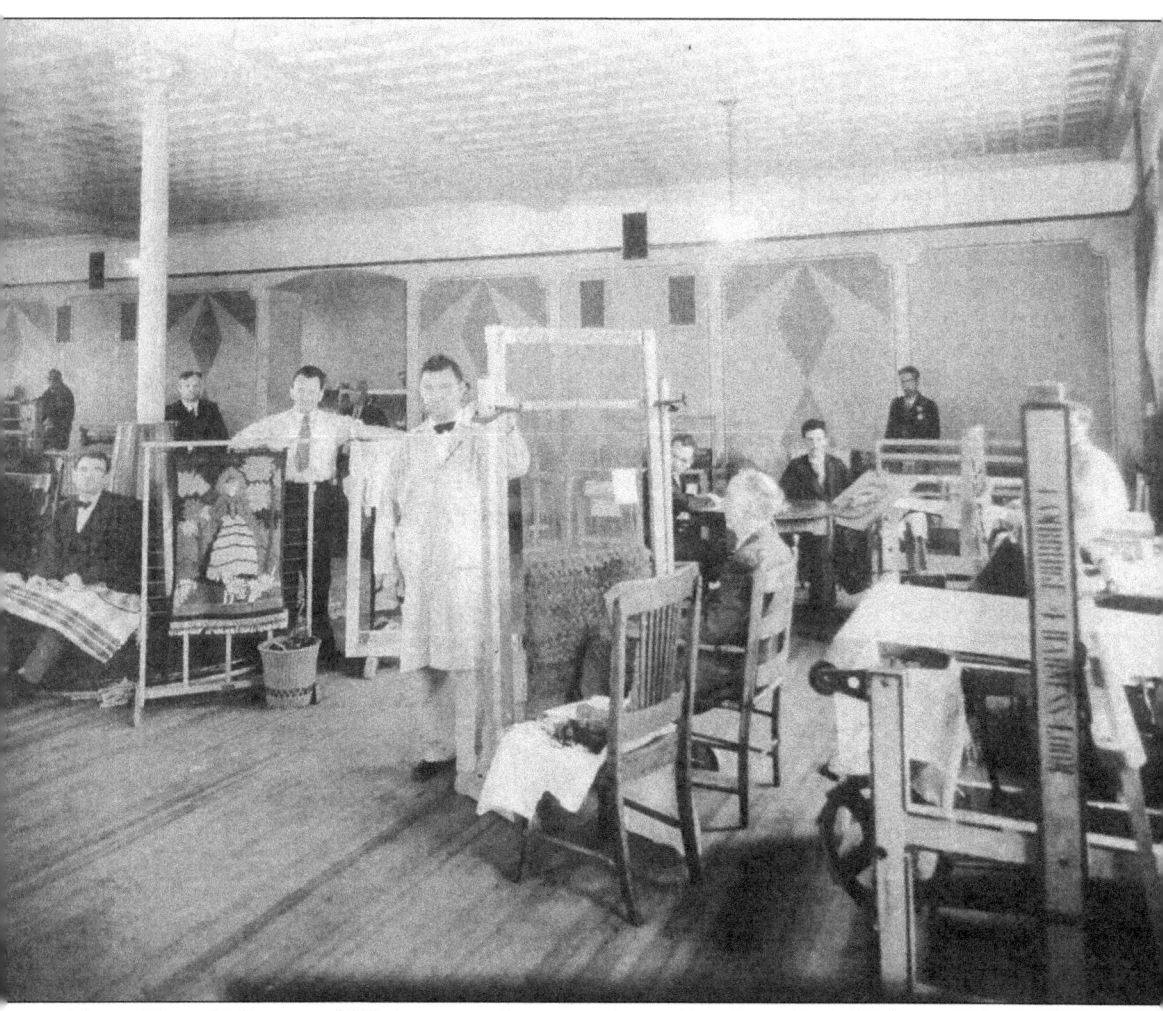

Also at Central Islip around 1920, a group of men are pictured in a large day hall. This unit, located in the Smith Group, was strictly for male inhabitants at that time. Steel-beam construction allowed for larger common areas uninterrupted by walls, as compared to older wood-frame buildings. At the time this photograph was taken, male staff were not permitted to work on female units. However, female staff could work on both male and female units. At center, a tall loom can be seen in use to weave a thick rug. At right is a loom used to weave sheets. Note the sharp dress of the men. Appearance was given a high priority; all individuals were fitted for tailored clothes upon arrival to the hospital.

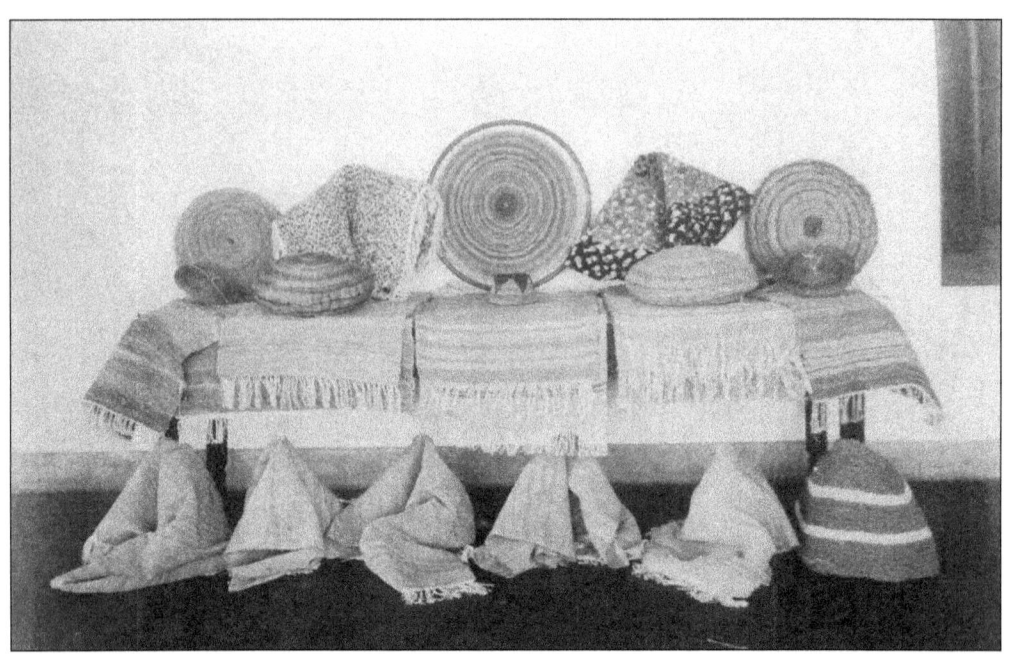

Above, completed rugs of various sizes and shapes are ready for sale or gallery display. Individuals earned wages for each article they produced upon its sale. Completed items were often a point of great pride for the patients, who labored to craft them. Below, a number of baskets woven out of reeds grown on the hospital grounds are displayed. Fine needlepoint designs can be observed as well. These items were displayed during an occupational therapy exhibit at Central Islip State Hospital around the 1920s.

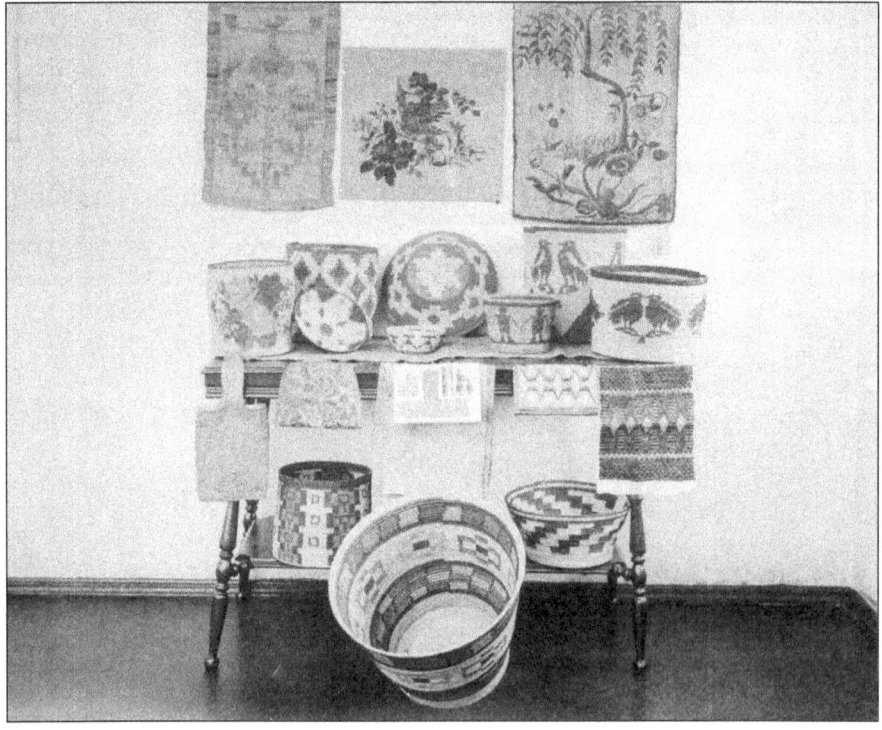

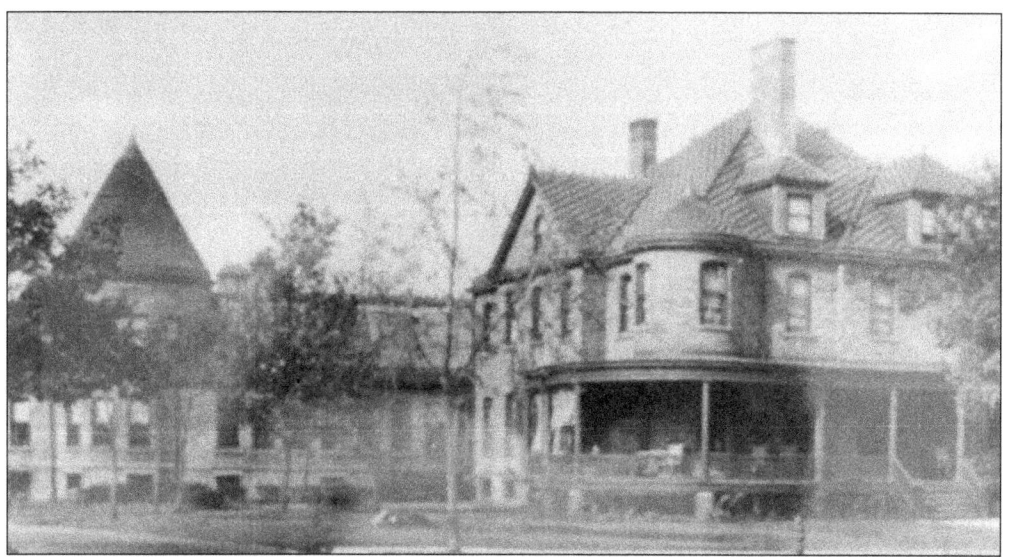

Common features at all the state hospitals were the ornate stone buildings and neatly manicured grounds. The early 1900s image above shows Group I at Kings Park State Hospital in its heyday. Group I provided combined living quarters, kitchen, and administration building and a hotel-like setting for those housed within. High ceilings, glass breezeways, heavy stone trim, and spacious quarters were grand elements of the building design. Below, a glass ceiling breezeway can be seen in use for a fall female social in 1915. The breezeways were designed to allow enough light to grow massive plants and extra space for patient use. (Both, courtesy of the Kings Park Heritage Museum.)

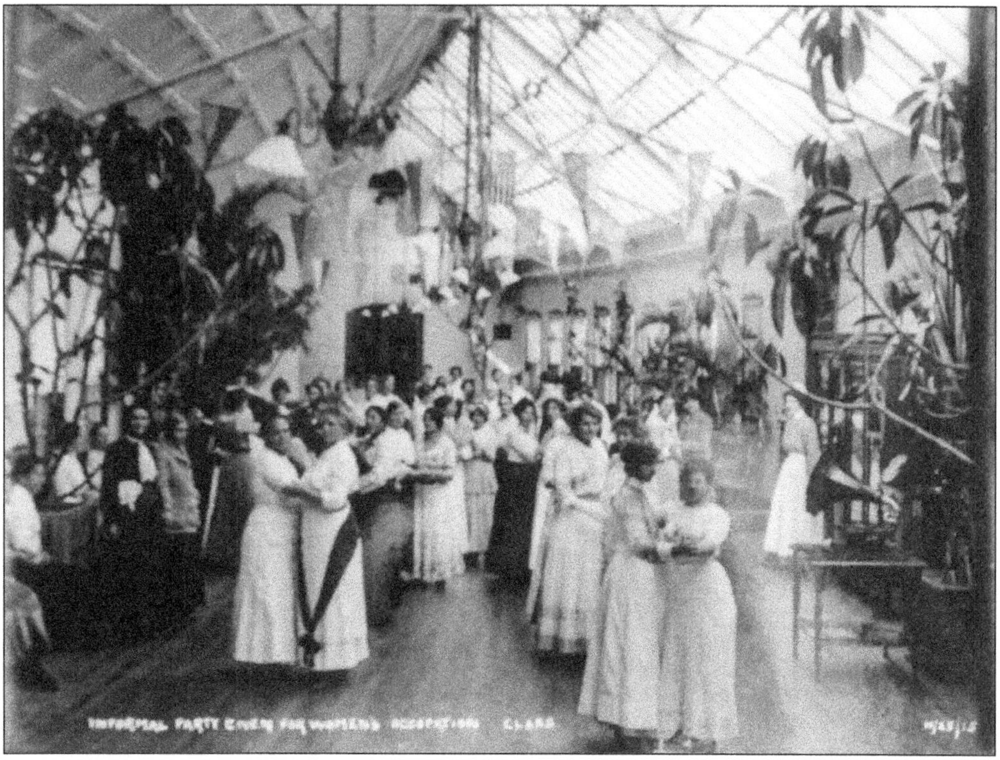

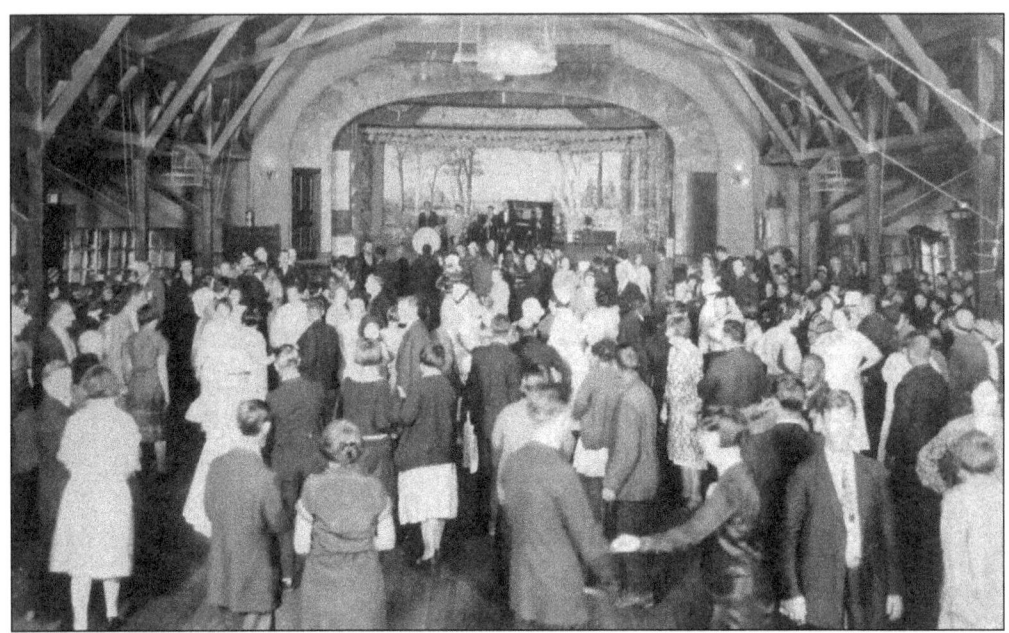

Dance socials were a long-standing tradition at the Long Island state hospitals. The evening would typically begin with a play or performance, followed by the dance. Musically inclined staff and patients would perform in the assembly halls. Above, men and women can be seen at a c. 1930s social at Central Islip State Hospital's first assembly hall. Below is Robbins Hall, the newer assembly hall at Central Islip, with practice for an upcoming dance in the 1950s taking place. At center is a baby grand piano.

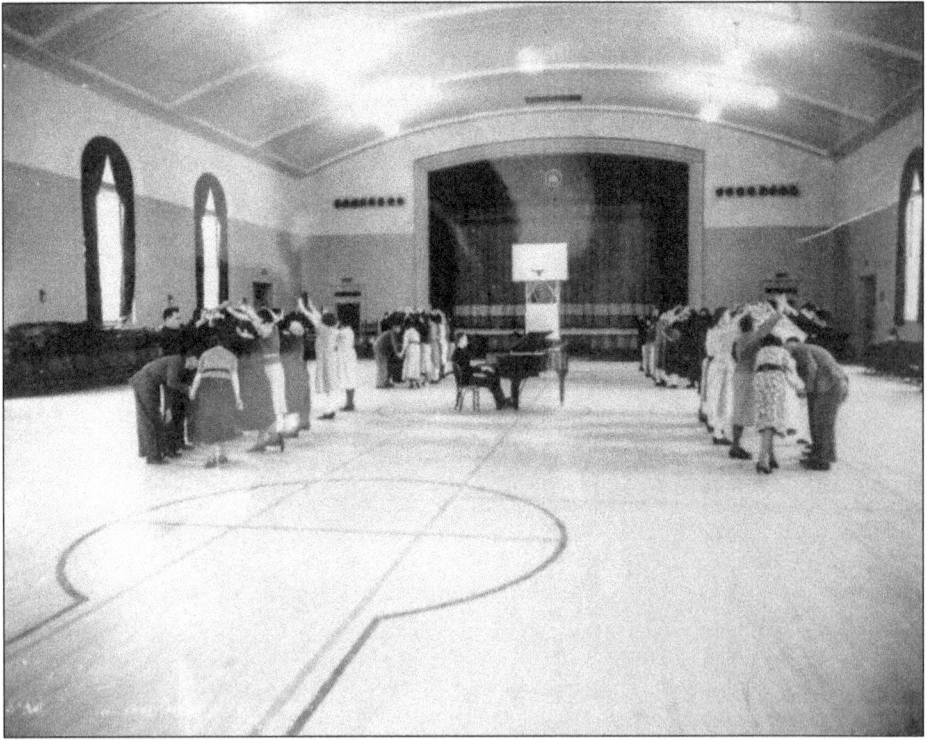

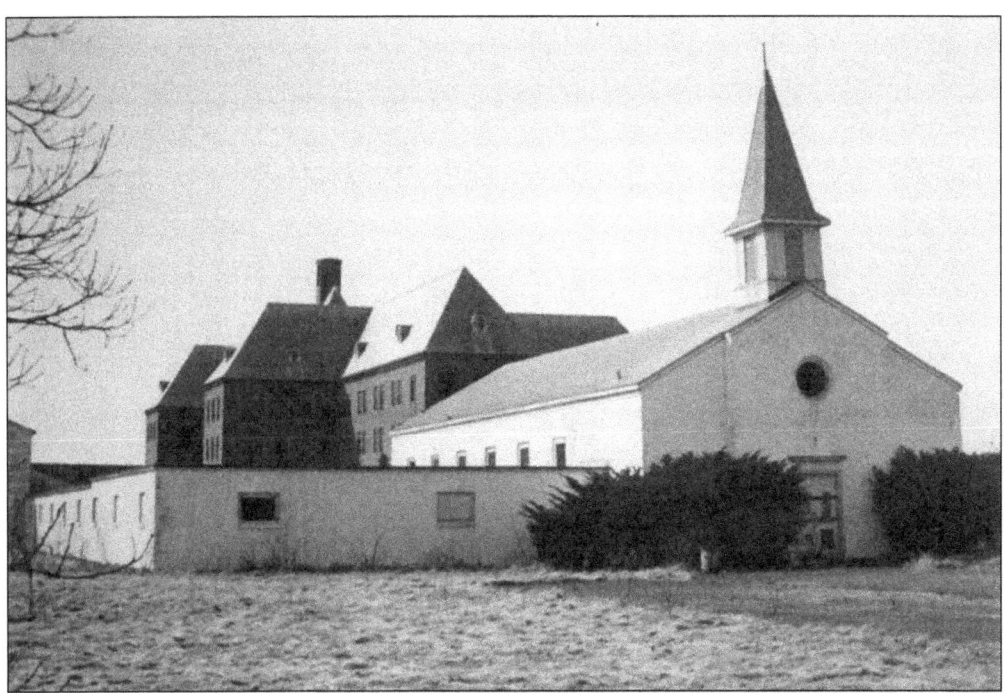

Religious services and counseling were made available to patients at the state hospitals. Both images were taken at the Edgewood State Hospital chapel. Edgewood had lofty plans when its construction began prior to World War II. It was to be completed on an even larger scale than the adjacent Pilgrim State Hospital campus; however, the project was federally funded, and the war effort drained the funds to complete the property. Only a handful of buildings were completed. The campus was turned over to Pilgrim State's control after World War II and remained open until the 1960s as a tuberculosis center. The photograph above was taken shortly after Edgewood closed. Note the massive main building in the background. The image below was taken in the chapel around Christmas in the early 1960s.

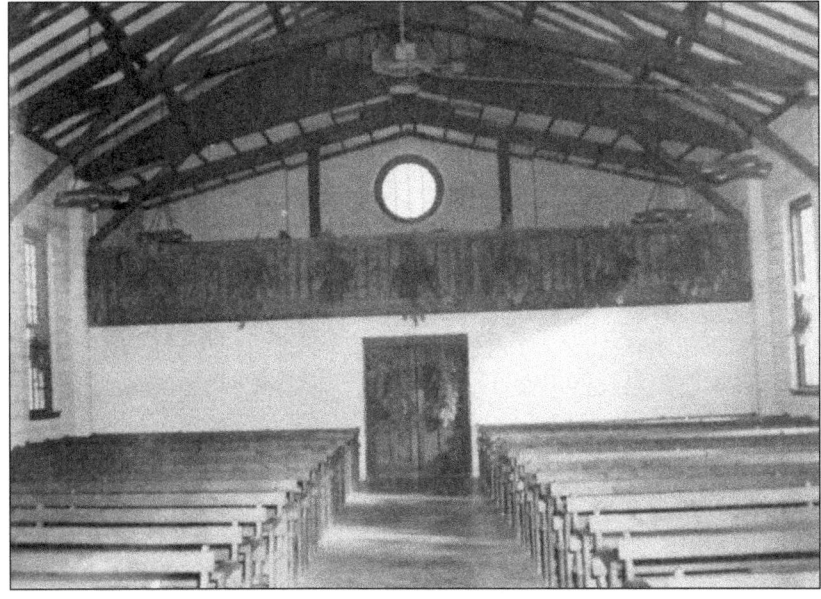

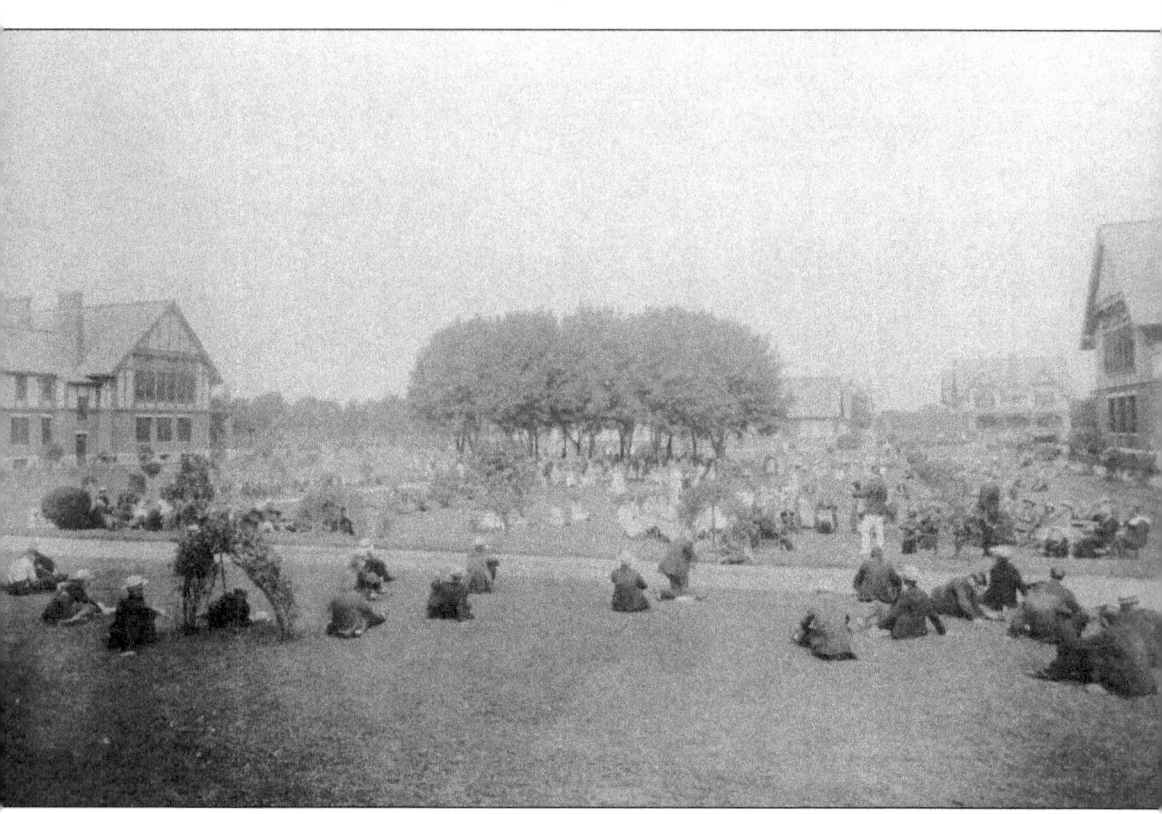

Contrary to a typical Hollywood stereotype, where patients were locked inside bland wards indefinitely, individuals at the state hospitals were out on the grounds or other unlocked areas regularly. The philosophy of moral therapy, which guided the care and treatment of patients for decades, was based on the blending of therapeutic activity with a serene environment. It is worth mentioning that for many decades before the advent of psychiatric medication, moral therapy led to the amelioration of symptoms and discharge of large numbers of patients from the state hospitals. On a spring day in a garden between the Smith Group buildings, patients are gathered at Central Islip State Hospital. In the right foreground, a band is playing. The tranquil atmosphere provided by the architecture and landscape one might find at an upscale resort of that period made for an exceptionally peaceful environment.

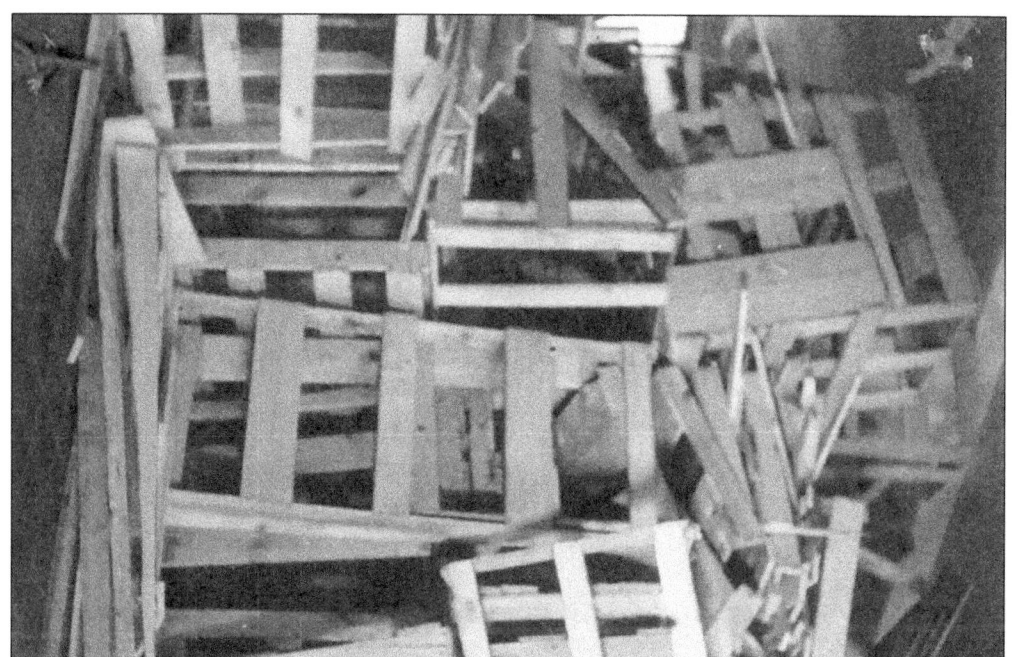

Few things went to waste at the state hospitals. The prudent practice of recycling materials kept the facilities' operating costs low. Above is a pile of scrap wood from pallets used to ship goods to the hospital. The occupational therapy (OT) department used these pallets for adaptive reuse into furniture, since pallets were often made of hardwoods. Many articles produced from the department were comprised of scrap materials, such as rugs made from old cloth scraps. The pallets were disassembled, and nails were removed so they could be resurfaced for reuse. Below, a finished cabinet made entirely of reclaimed lumber is on proud display at Pilgrim State Hospital at a 1930s OT fair.

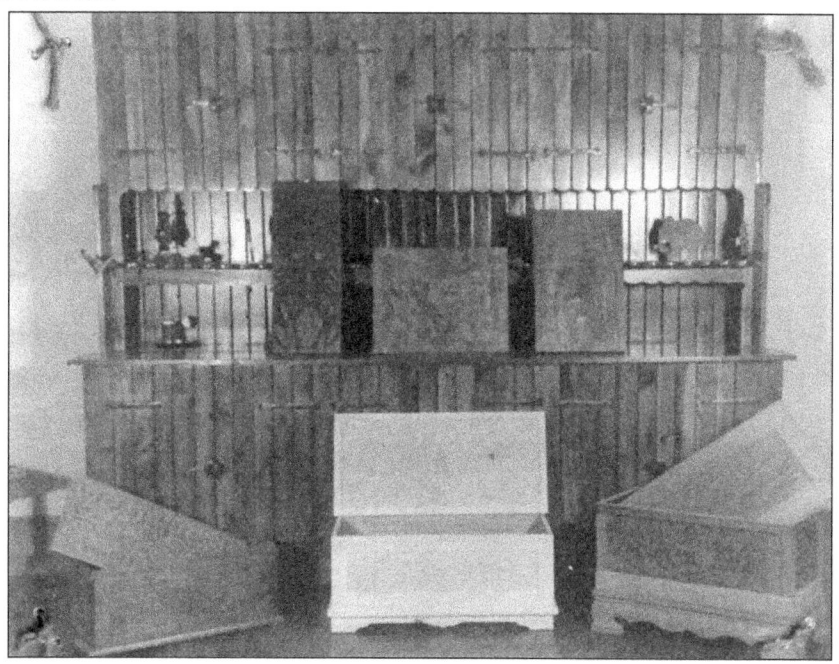

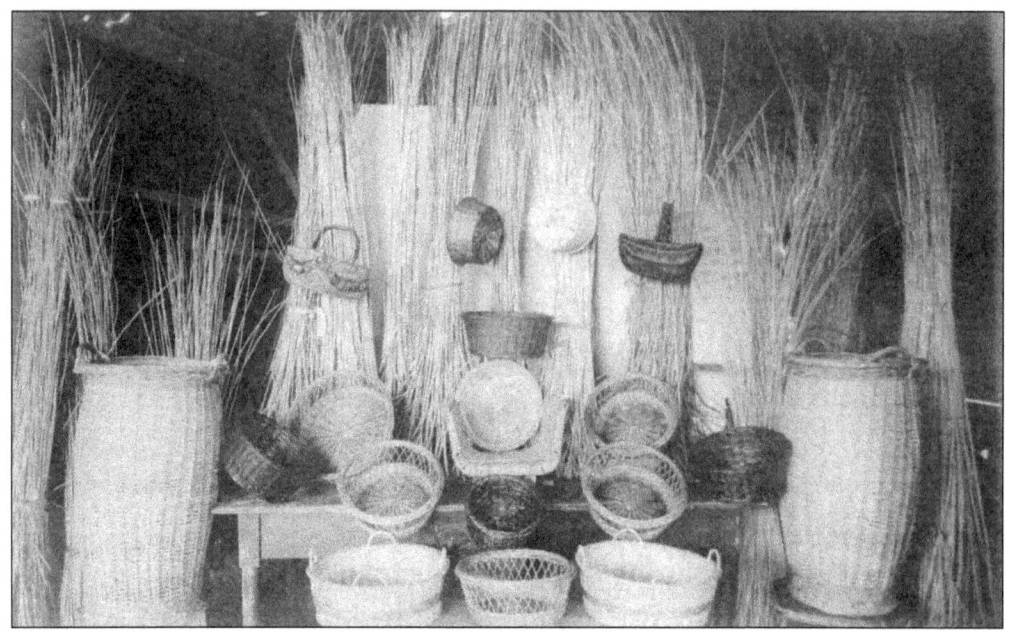

Some tasks assigned to patients by the activities staff differed between sexes. Basket weaving was predominantly a male activity, whereas sewing was predominantly female. Above are baskets weaved by male patients at Central Islip State Hospital. Bundles of reeds harvested from the grounds are seen. From these reeds, the baskets were woven at virtually no cost. Below is a 1930s occupational therapy exhibit at Central Islip, with various articles produced by patients on display. At center is a table of assorted handcrafted figurines made in the toy shop.

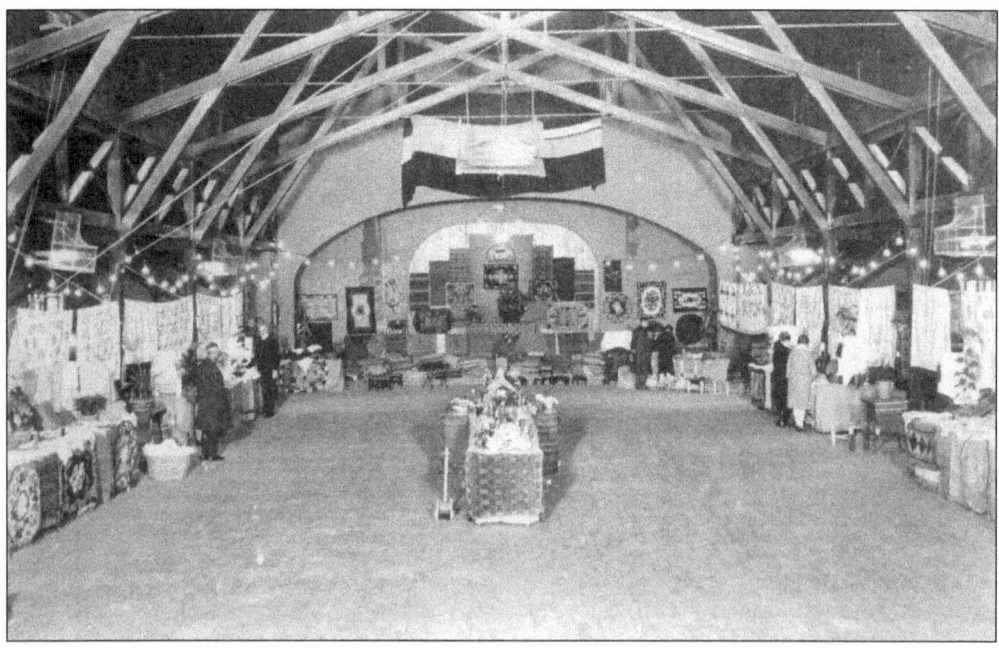

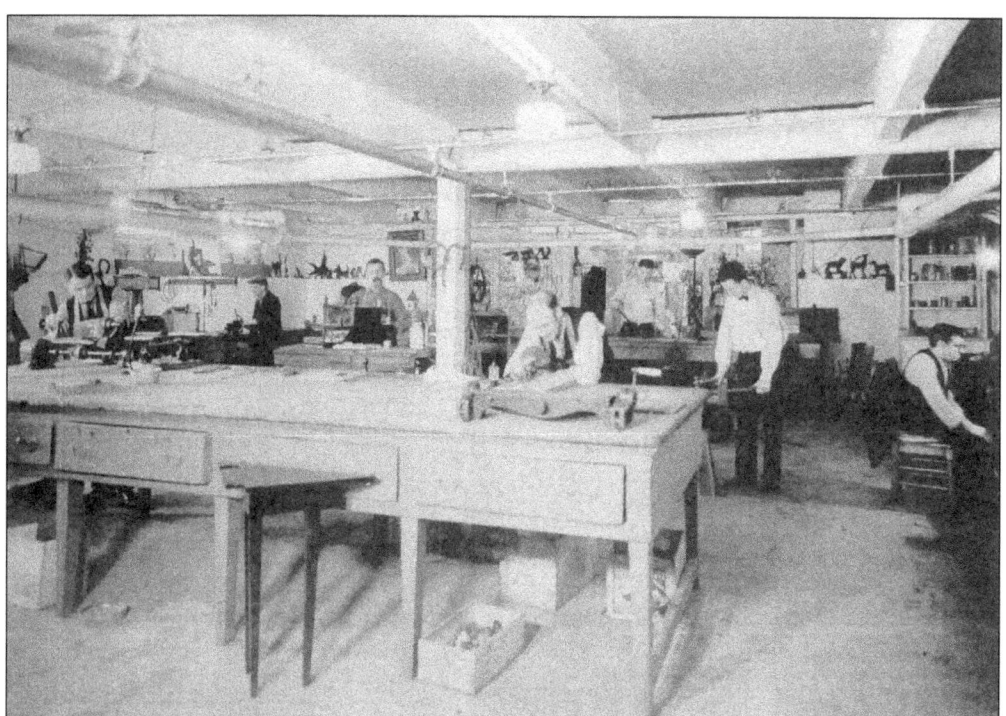

The state hospitals were nearly fully autonomous for the majority of their operating years. Food, furniture, and other necessities were not the only items produced onsite—recreation articles were also made. Above, at Central Islip State Hospital, a group of men work in a shop dedicated to toy making. The toys were purchased by staff or patients at sales and distributed to all areas of the hospital where they were age appropriate to be enjoyed by patients. Below, at Central Islip, a table of toys is displayed at an OT fair around the 1930s.

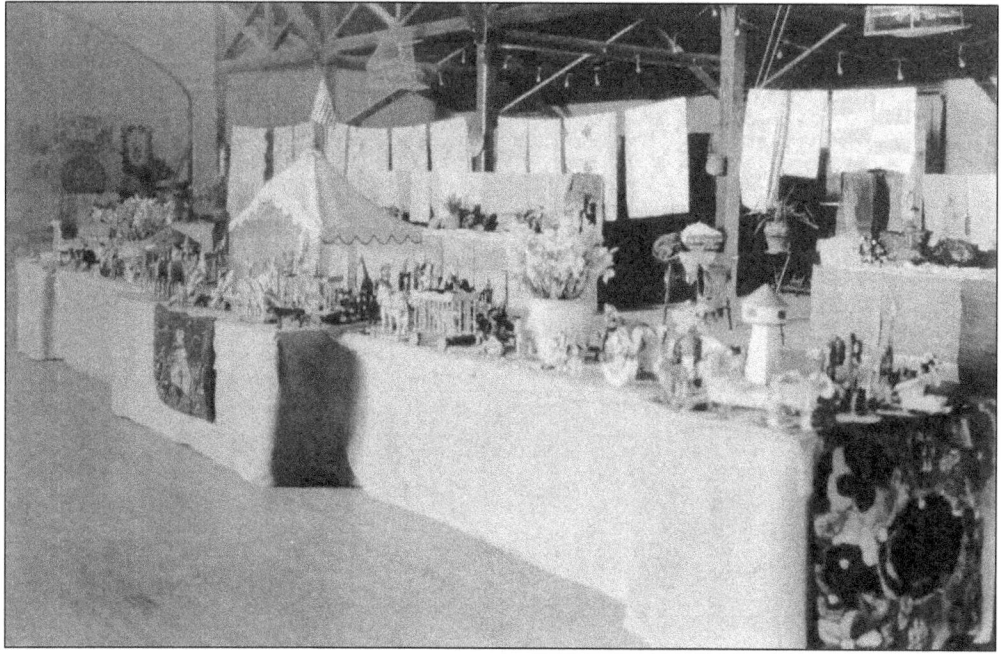

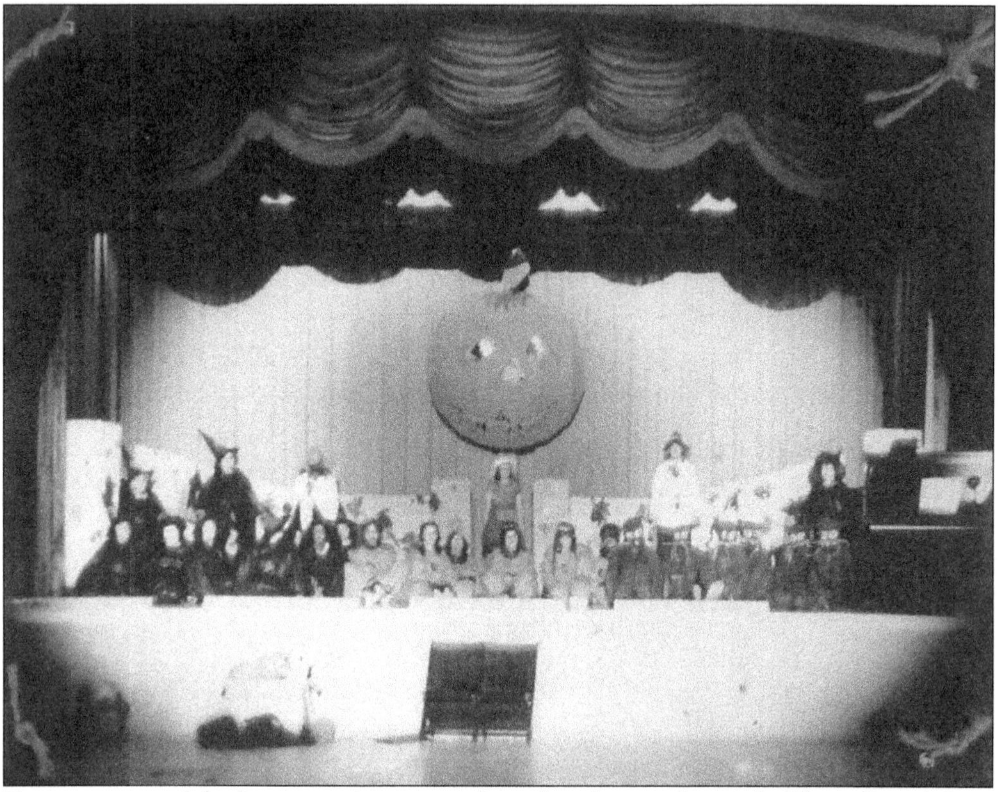

Plays were part of the live entertainment performed at the state hospitals. They allowed those who had artistic talent an opportunity to craft scenery and props for use in the show. Theater allowed patients to explore new talent as well as bring cheer to the facility. The cast seen here was photographed at Pilgrim State Hospital around Halloween.

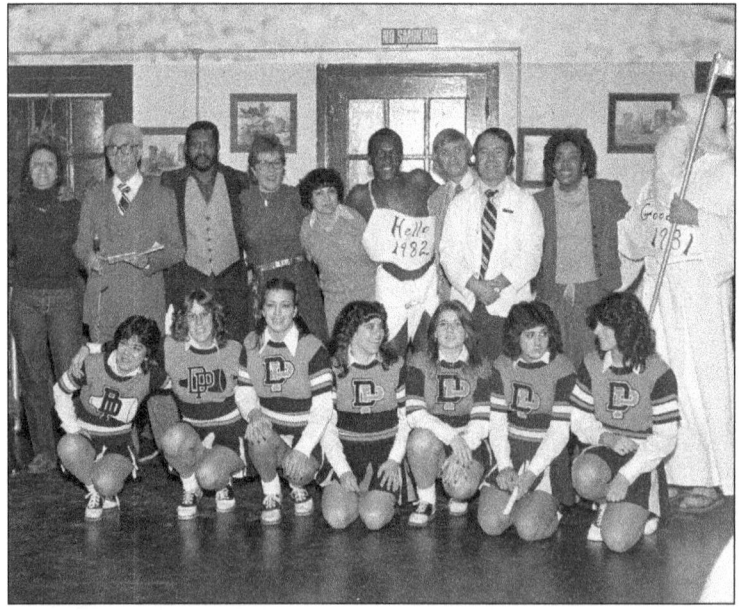

The local high schools have visited Pilgrim State Hospital around the holidays for many decades, singing Christmas carols and even performing a kick line. This group of Deer Park High School cheerleaders poses with hospital staff after spreading some holiday cheer in 1981.

For children who resided at the state hospitals, not being enrolled in a typical school with their peers was hard. To aid in transforming the hospital environment, extra care was taken in considering the type and quality of recreation for children. In the 1960s, this puppet play for children was put on in Building 26, the assembly hall at Pilgrim State Hospital.

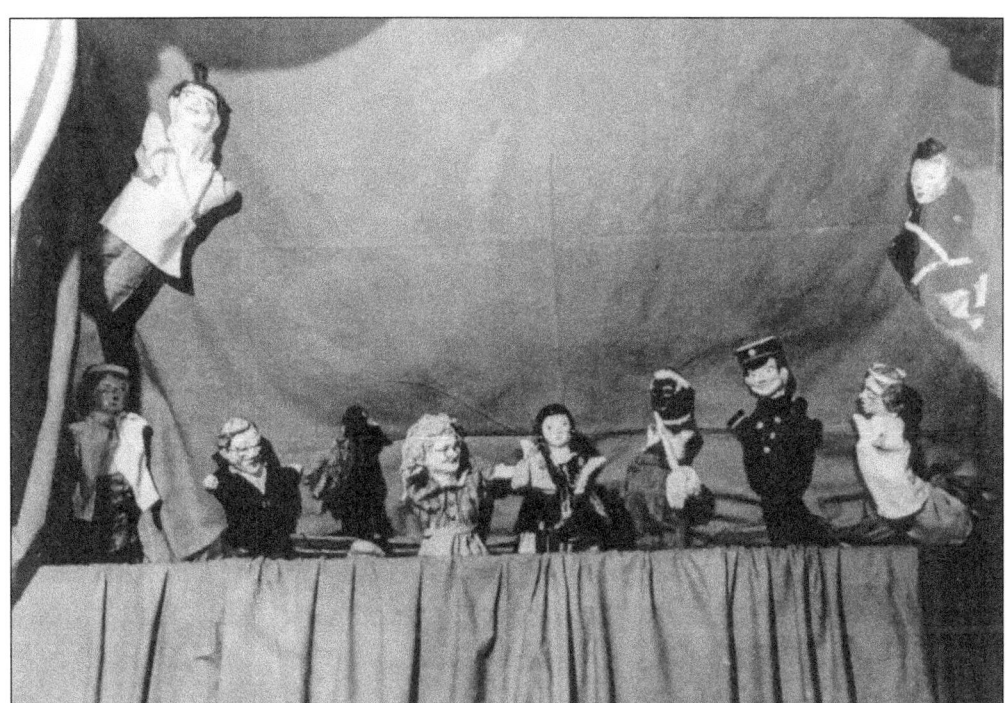

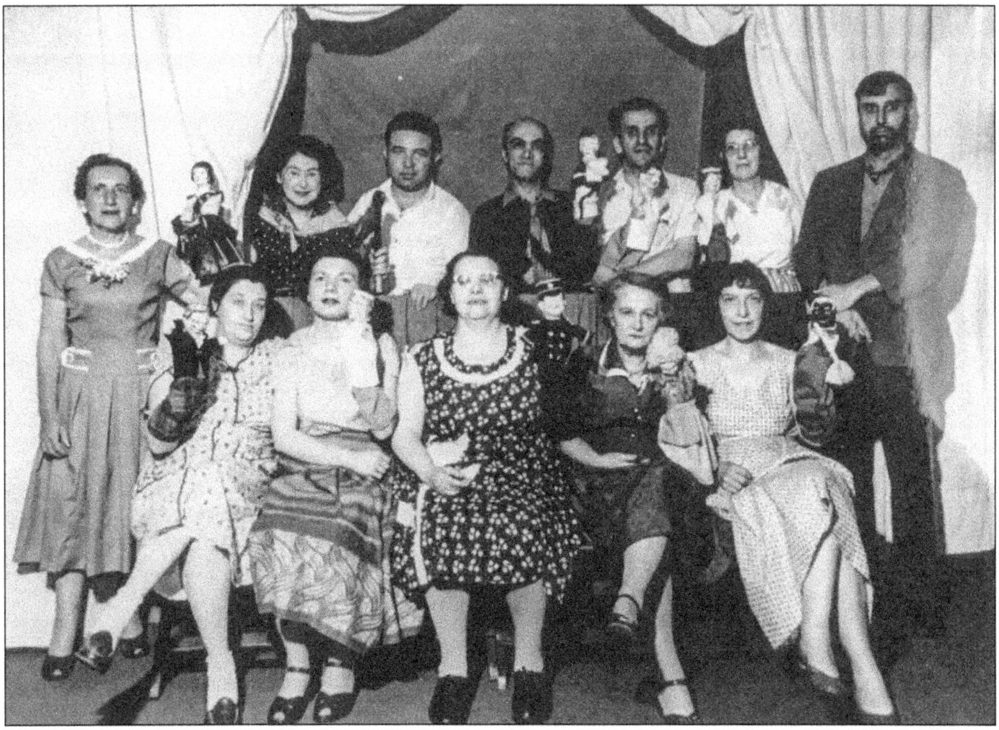

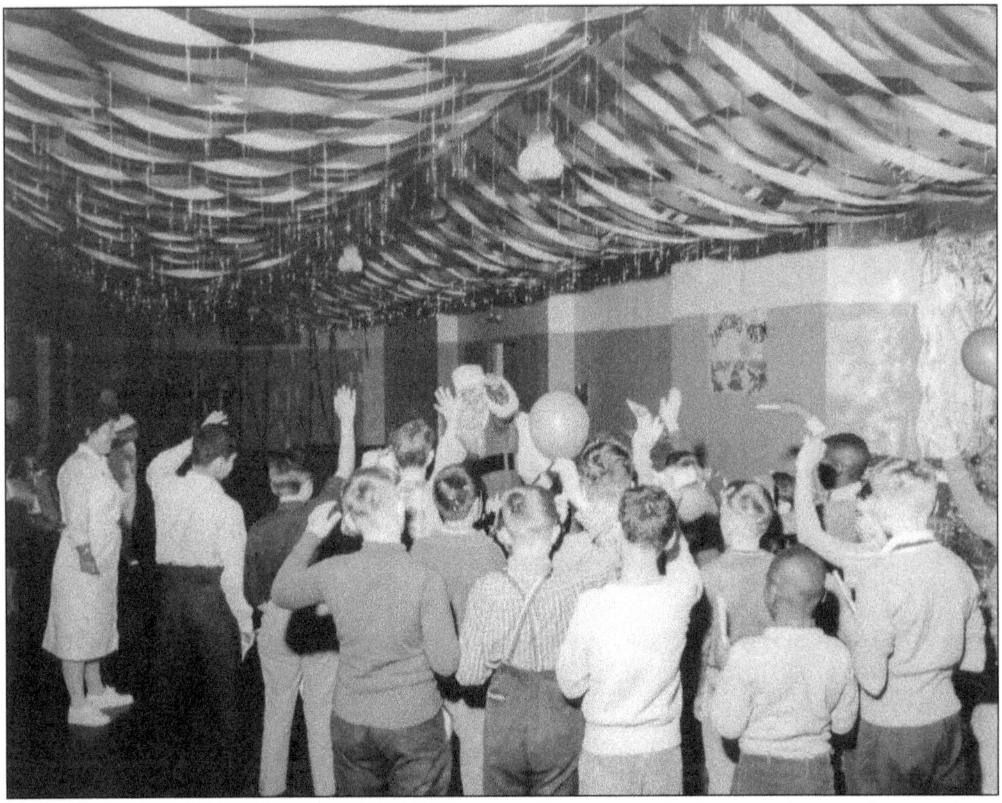

The hallway of the children's unit in Building 127/128 at Central Islip State Hospital is seen here in the 1950s. The streamers hung from the ceiling were placed by the recreation department for Christmas. Specialty items were often added to the menu to lift spirits during the holidays. These children were off to a Christmas celebration in the adjoining dining hall.

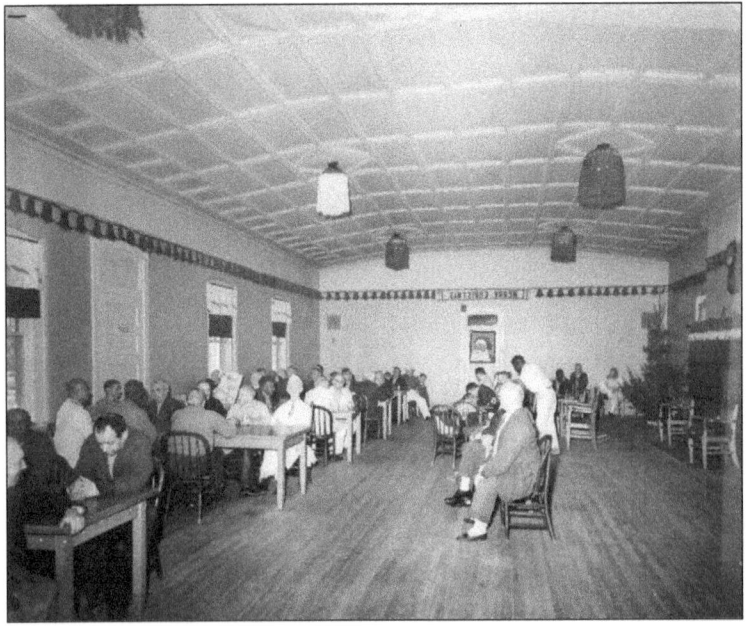

At Central Islip State Hospital during Christmas, men socialize on a crowded ward in a living unit on the grounds. A Christmas tree can be seen in the rear at right.

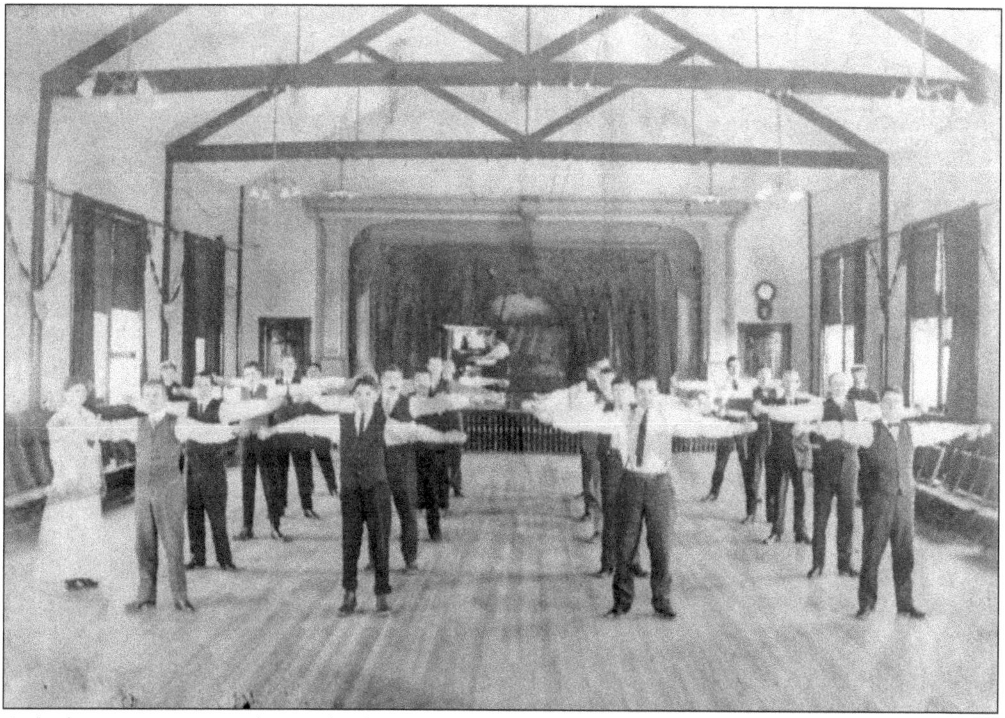

Calisthenics was a popular method of exercise in the 1920s when these photographs were taken at Kings Park State Hospital. Men gathered in the recreation building for group exercise. Staff and patients both routinely exercised while living at the hospitals. A sedentary lifestyle was not encouraged. Sports and fitness were highly regarded as critical for promoting general welfare. Contrary to the misconception that physical fitness was a trend of the 21st century, exercise and health awareness were linchpins of the previous centuries as well. (Both, courtesy of the Kings Park Heritage Museum.)

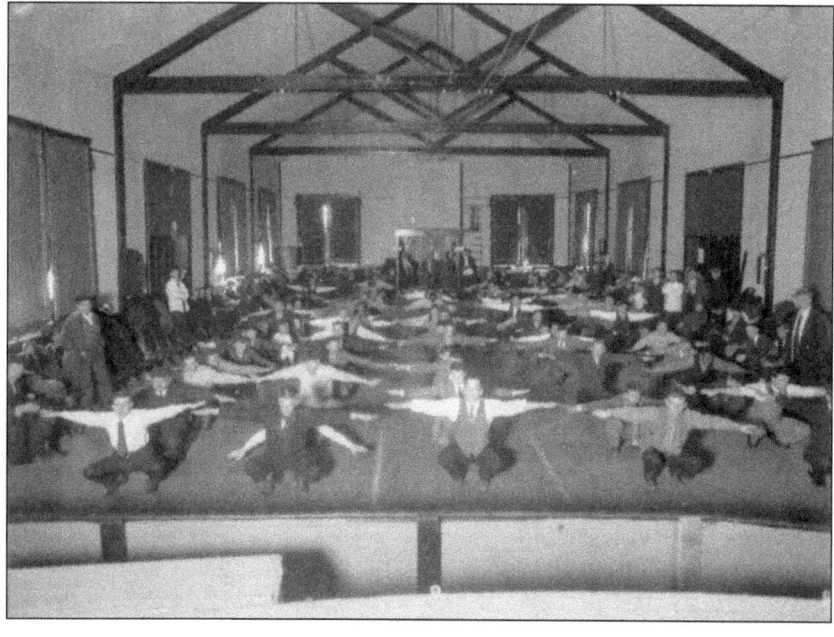

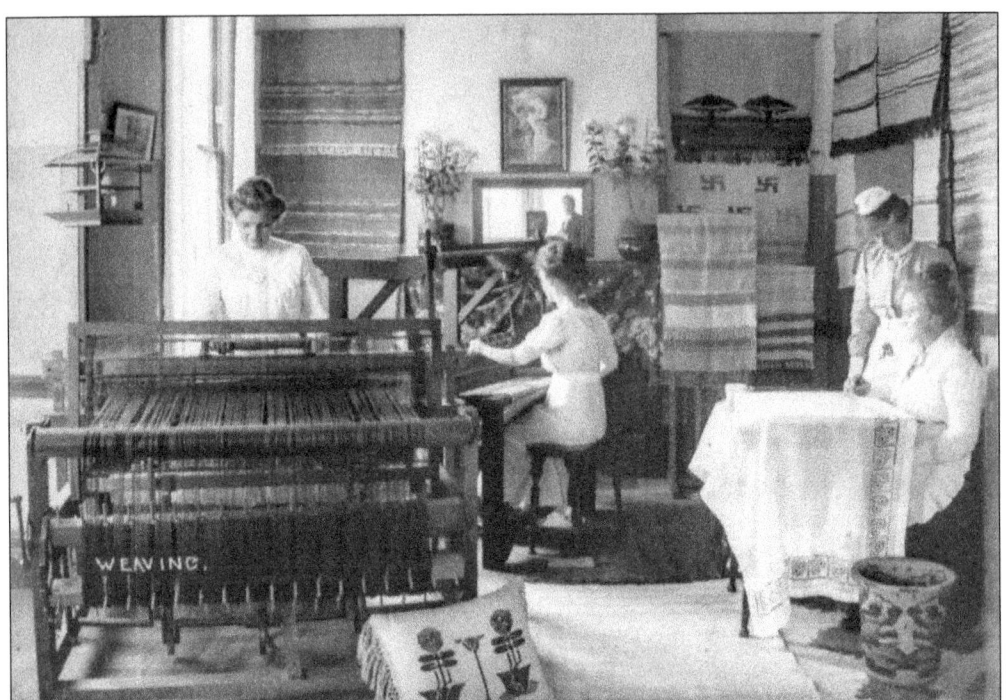

Looms provided a variety of textiles woven from yarn or thread at a low cost. The wooden looms created stock for clothing, rugs, and other products. From cloth woven on the grounds, quality clothing and uniforms could be custom tailored to an individual at low cost. In these photographs taken at Kings Park State Hospital in the 1920s, women can be seen in an occupational therapy class. Finished decorative cloths and rugs hang on the walls. Note the intricate details in the quilts and tablecloths. (Both, courtesy of the Kings Park Heritage Museum.)

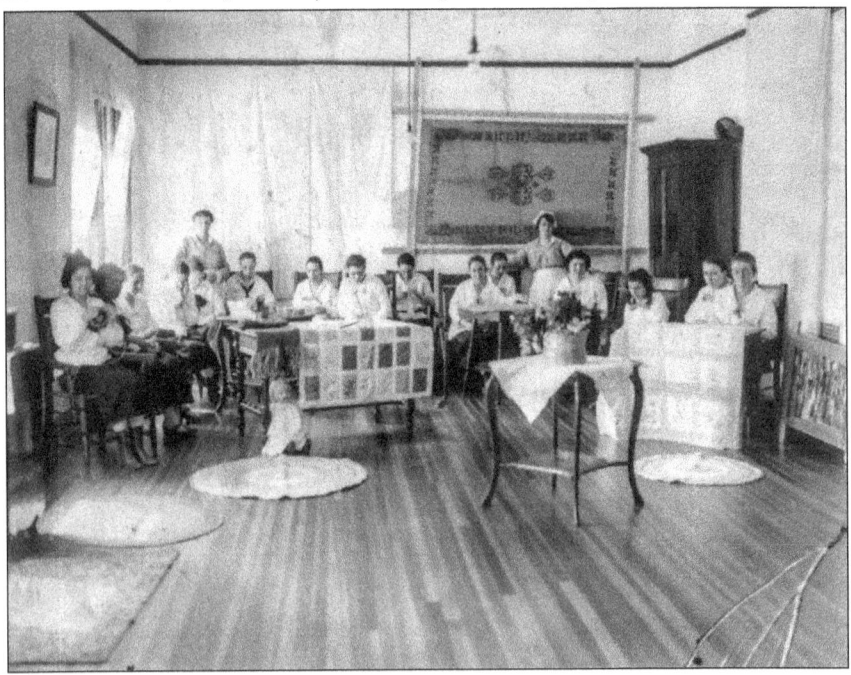

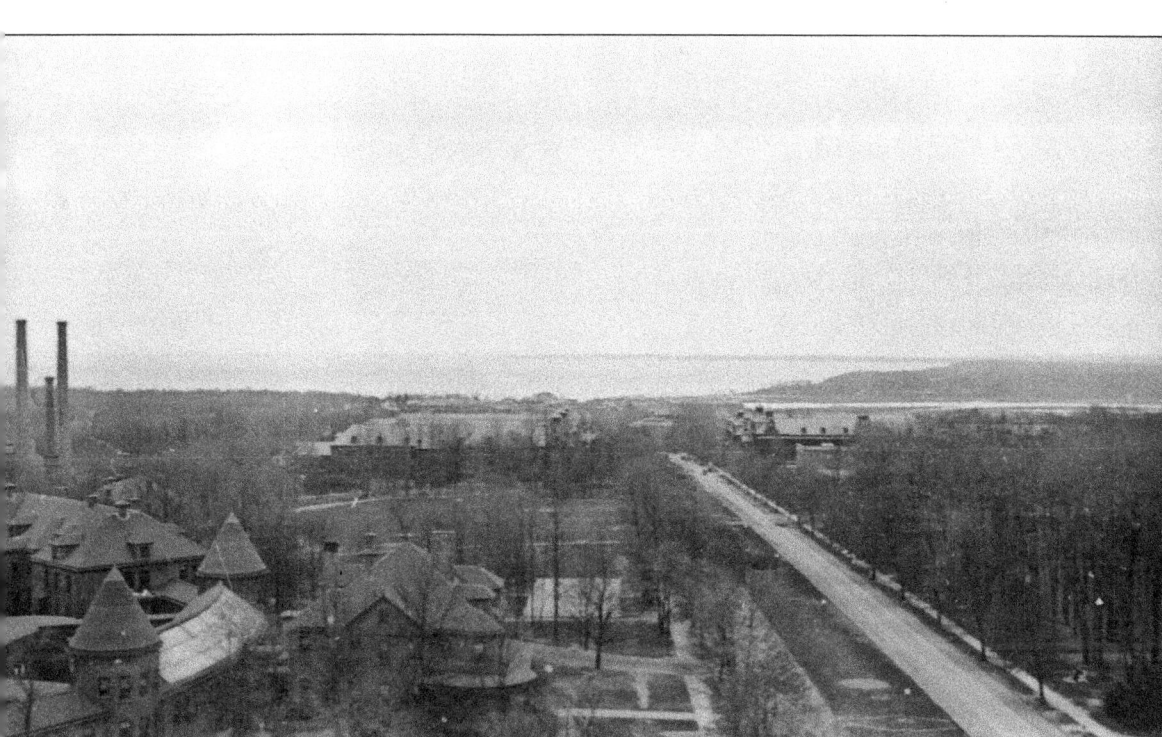

This early-20th-century look at the grounds of Kings Park State Hospital gives a sense of its once mammoth size. In the view looking from the boulevard down to Long Island Sound, a few notable structures can be seen. To the left, three smokestacks tower up from the first and second powerhouses built on the property. The crescent moon shape of Group I, with its gothic stonework, is prominent. Farther down the beech tree–lined boulevard, Buildings A, B, C, and D can be seen across the street from one another.

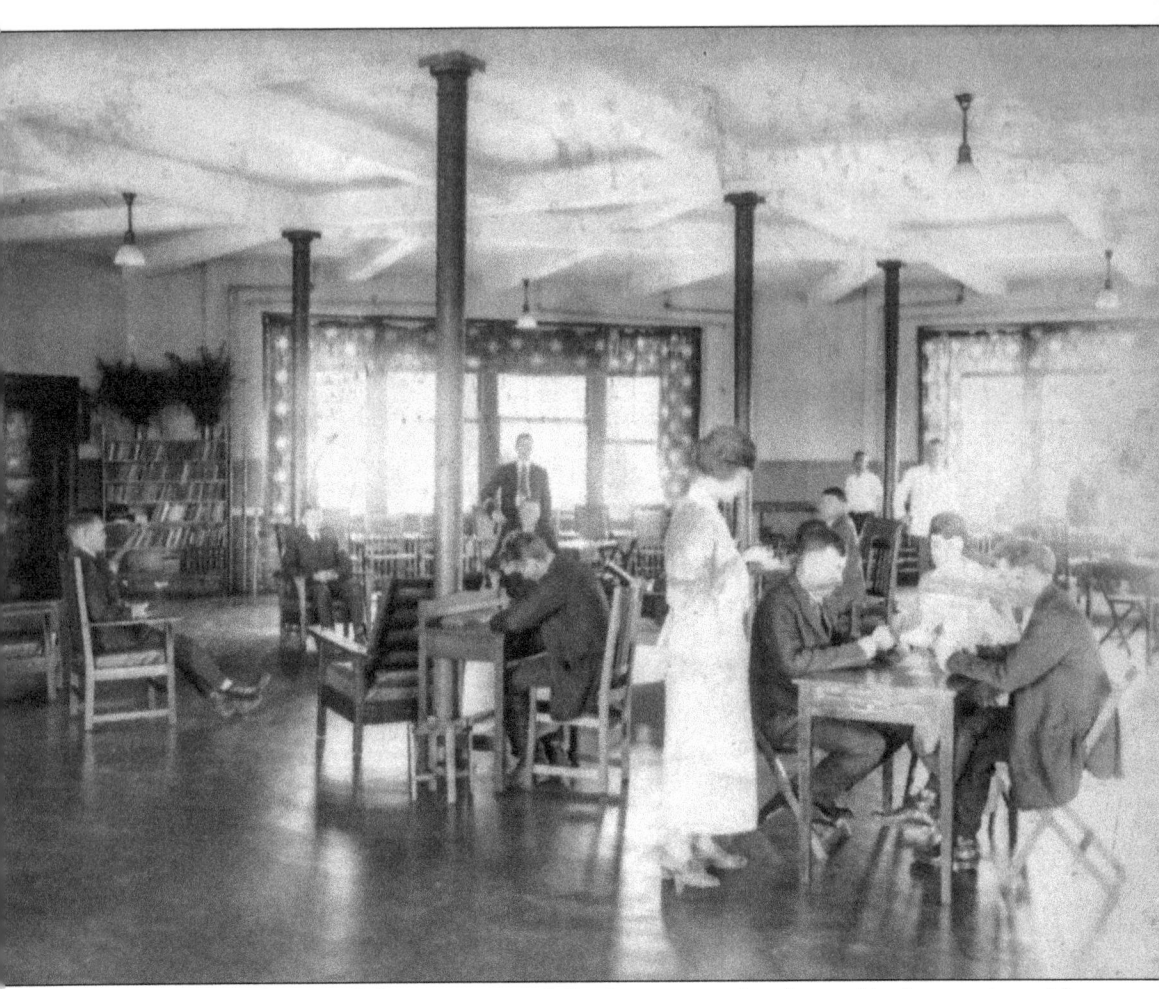

For many in the age of electronics, it is difficult to comprehend a world of recreation without modern devices. Here, a variety of leisure-time activities are captured in this photograph taken in one of the wards of Group I at Kings Park State Hospital. A game of cards between male and female occupational therapy aides is taking place at right. At center, a man writes a letter, and behind him, men sit in leather upholstered chairs. In the rear, hospital attendants can be seen in their white shirts. The tall ceilings are adorned with decorative glass lighting globes. Large windows allow sunlight to pour in. Oak furniture and a tall bookcase fill the room. These furnishings were nearly identical to those found at an elegant social club of the day. (Courtesy of the Kings Park Heritage Museum.)

The occupational therapy department changed locations over the course of its existence at Kings Park State Hospital. In this image taken in the 1930s, the OT office was located in Group I. Articles from talented patients adorn the room to serve as a living museum of sorts for those who visited the office. A uniformed female OT worker can be seen in the background. (Courtesy of the Kings Park Heritage Museum.)

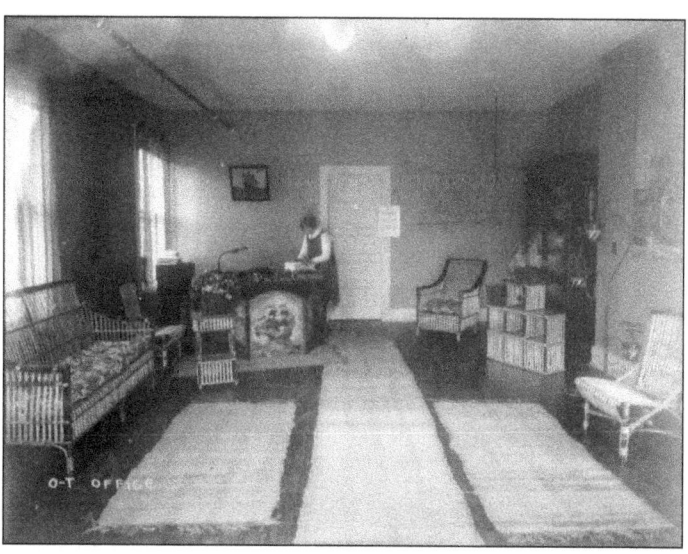

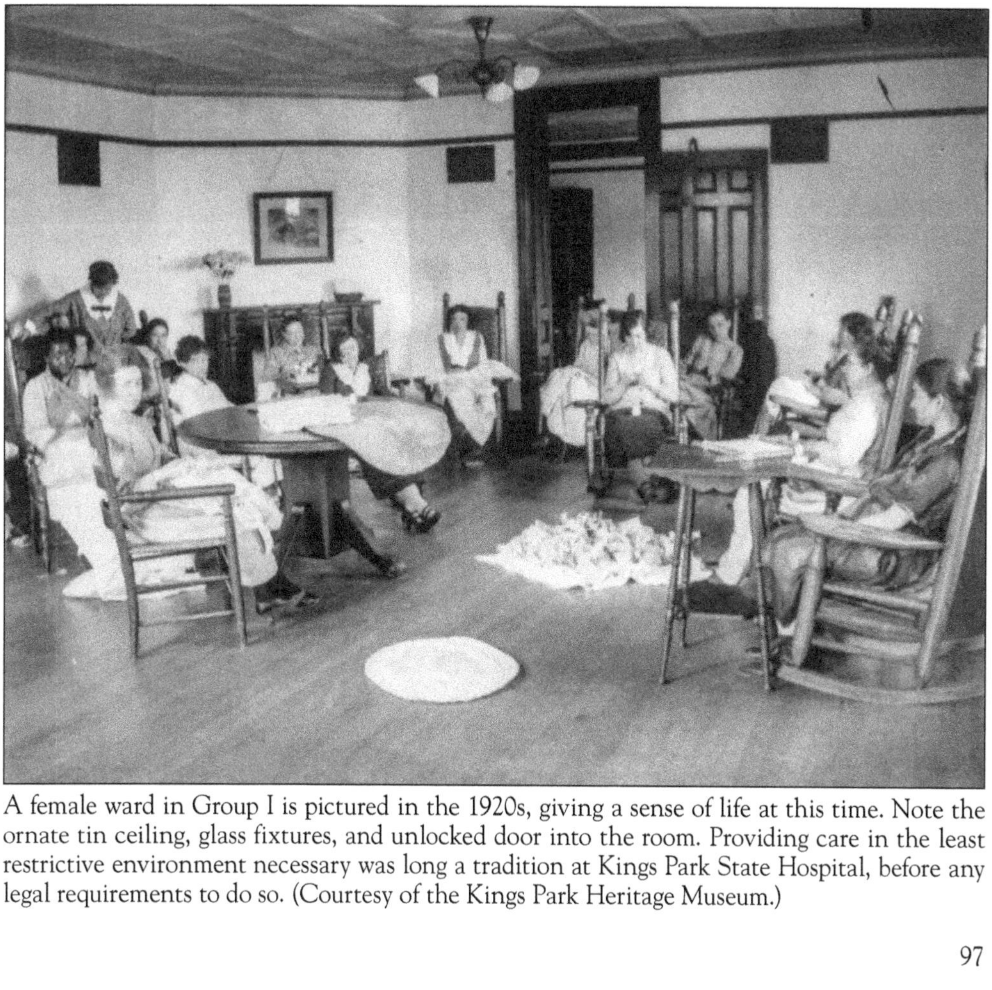

A female ward in Group I is pictured in the 1920s, giving a sense of life at this time. Note the ornate tin ceiling, glass fixtures, and unlocked door into the room. Providing care in the least restrictive environment necessary was long a tradition at Kings Park State Hospital, before any legal requirements to do so. (Courtesy of the Kings Park Heritage Museum.)

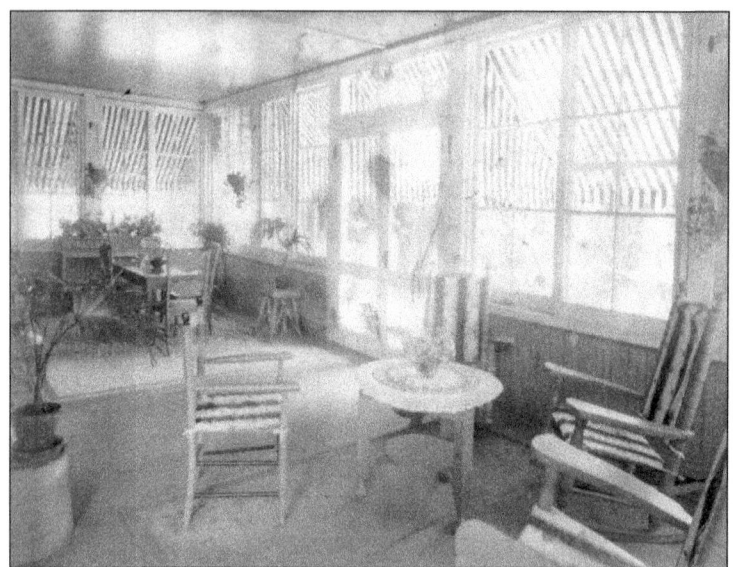

Porches were enclosed in glass to provide all-season rooms for staff and patients. This allowed for the year-round ability to keep plants growing. Horticulture was a popular pastime at Kings Park State Hospital. The plants seen here contributed to a homely setting. (Courtesy of the Kings Park Heritage Museum.)

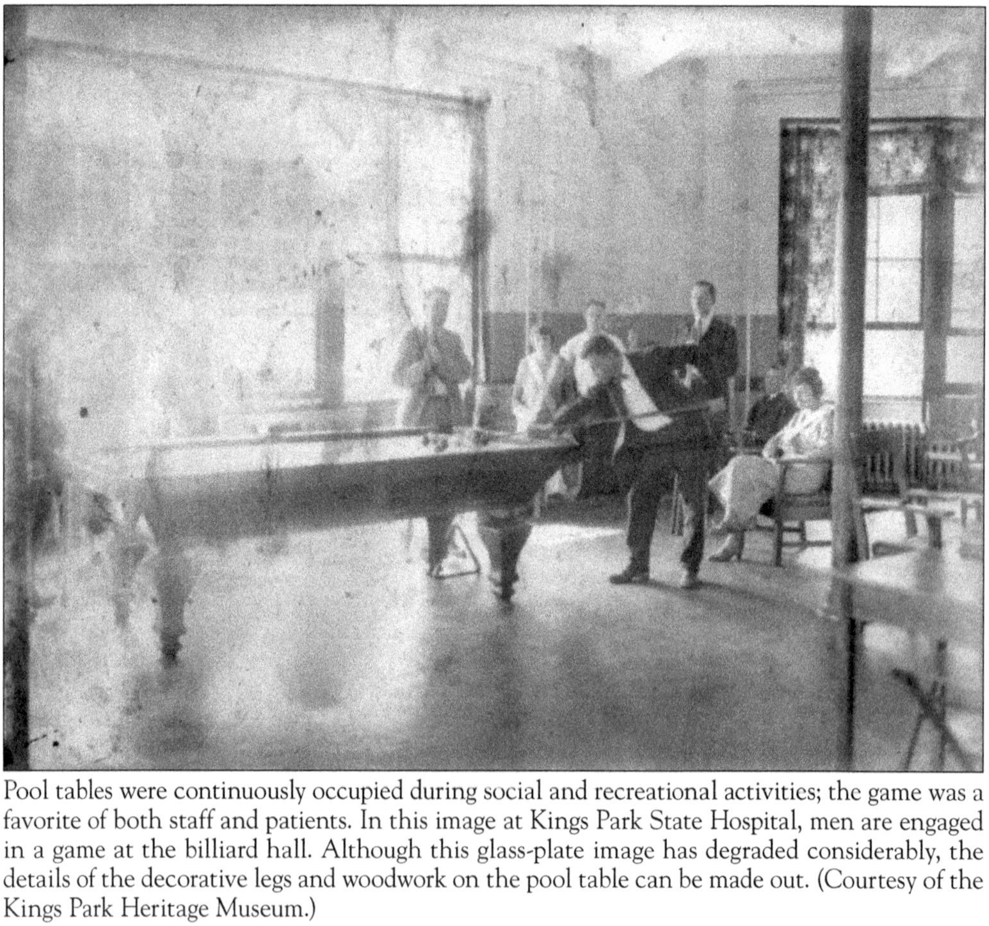

Pool tables were continuously occupied during social and recreational activities; the game was a favorite of both staff and patients. In this image at Kings Park State Hospital, men are engaged in a game at the billiard hall. Although this glass-plate image has degraded considerably, the details of the decorative legs and woodwork on the pool table can be made out. (Courtesy of the Kings Park Heritage Museum.)

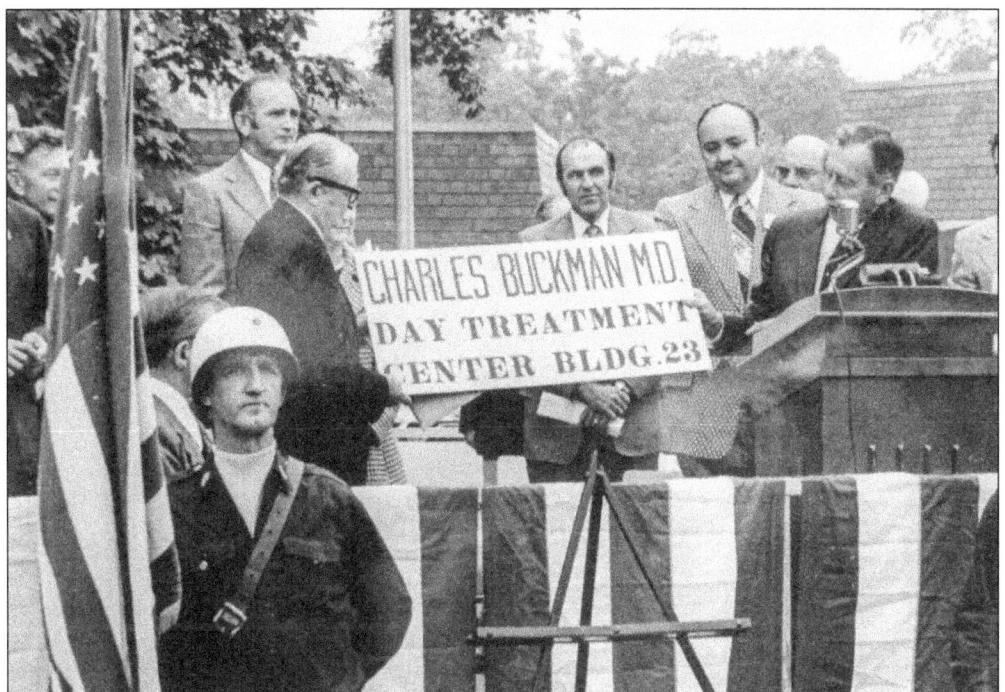

Occupational therapy split into OT and Therapeutic Recreation after World War II, resulting in steady job growth. By the 1960s, psychiatric rehabilitation was not only a new branch of service delivery to prepare patients for gainful employment in society, it also became the guiding care model for institutions until recent times. Operating in group space was practical and homogenous to the three branches of treatment. As a result, Building 23, also known as the rehab center, was built at Kings Park State Hospital in 1970 to provide modern space to run OT, rehabilitation, and recreation groups. Above is the dedication of Building 23's to Dr. Charles Buckman, a director of Kings Park. Below in the background, a poster advertising an art show in the 1970s is visible.

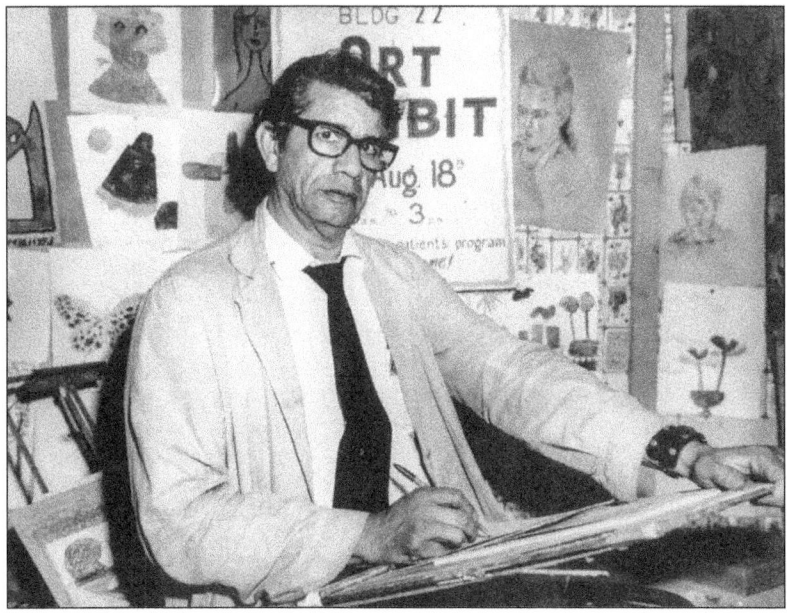

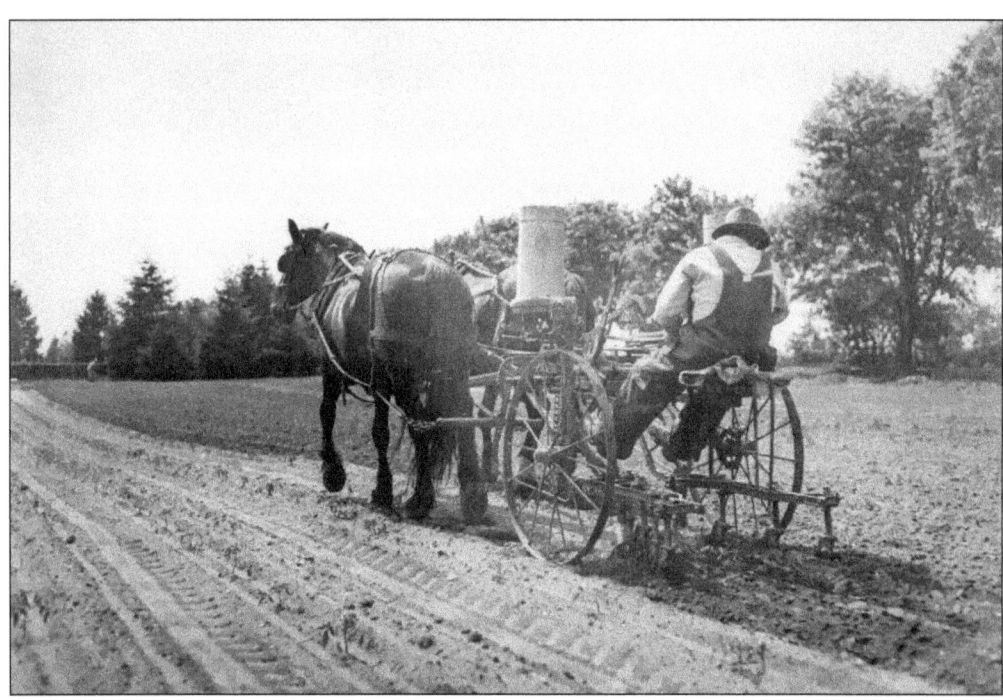

Prior to the automobile or steam engine, horses were a staple of life. At Kings Park State Hospital, horses were a familiar sight until the 1940s, when they were largely replaced by trucks and machines with gas engines. Above, a pair of horses are plowing the sandy farmland alongside Kings Park Boulevard. This would become the location of the final buildings constructed and left in operation at Kings Park. Below, in a winter scene during the 1930s, a horse is dragging a snow plow on the sidewalk adjacent to the tree-lined Boulevard at Kings Park.

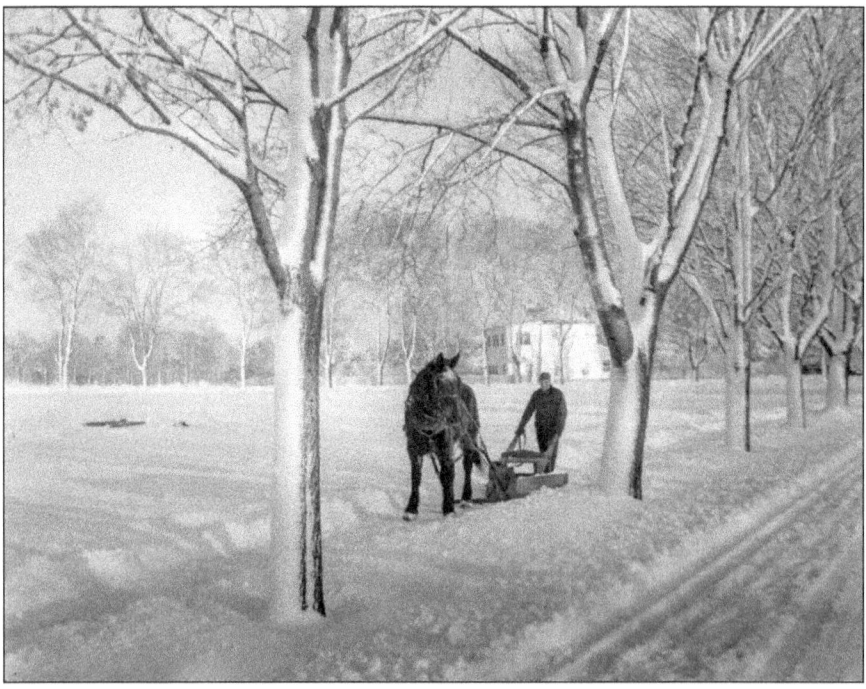

Until the 1970s, when the hospitals began to decrease the production of goods, quality textiles were hand-produced on site. Here, in a sewing room at Central Islip State Hospital, women work together on various projects. This was an opportunity for those who were not skilled to learn a trade.

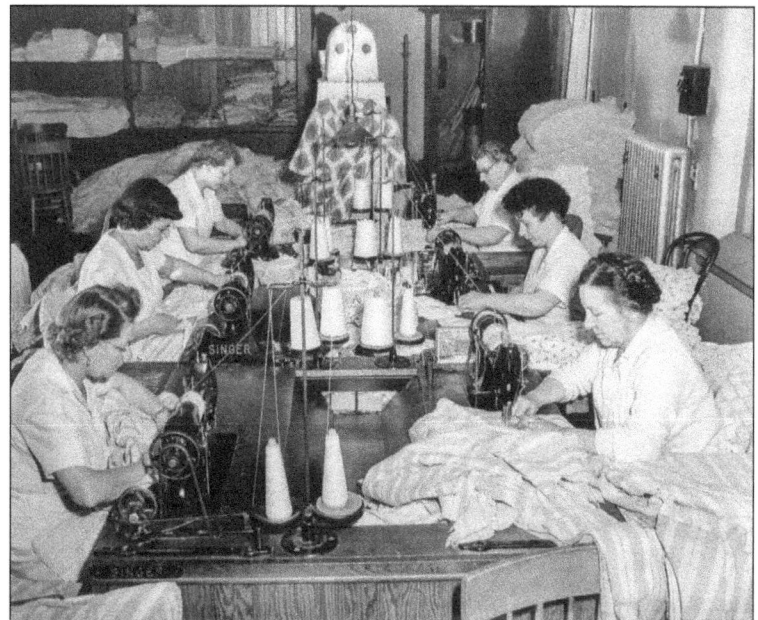

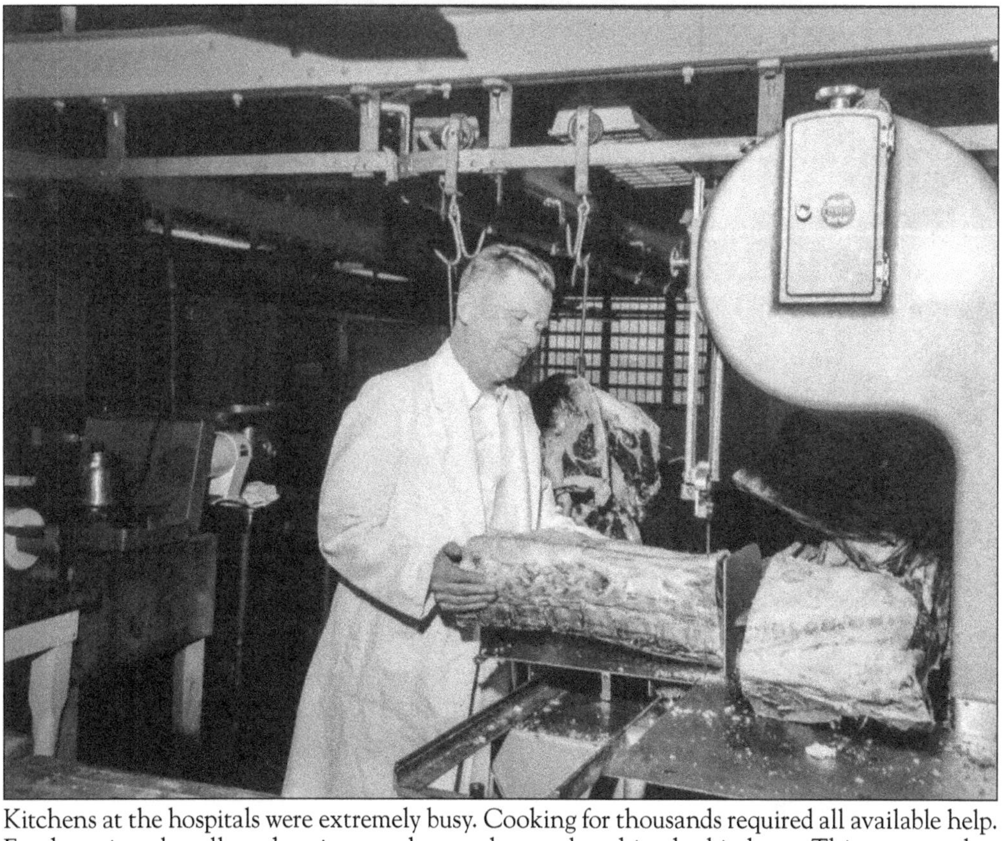

Kitchens at the hospitals were extremely busy. Cooking for thousands required all available help. Food service also allowed patient workers to be employed in the kitchens. This was another employable skill for patients to use after discharge. At Central Islip State Hospital, a man uses a bandsaw to cut portions of beef for roasting.

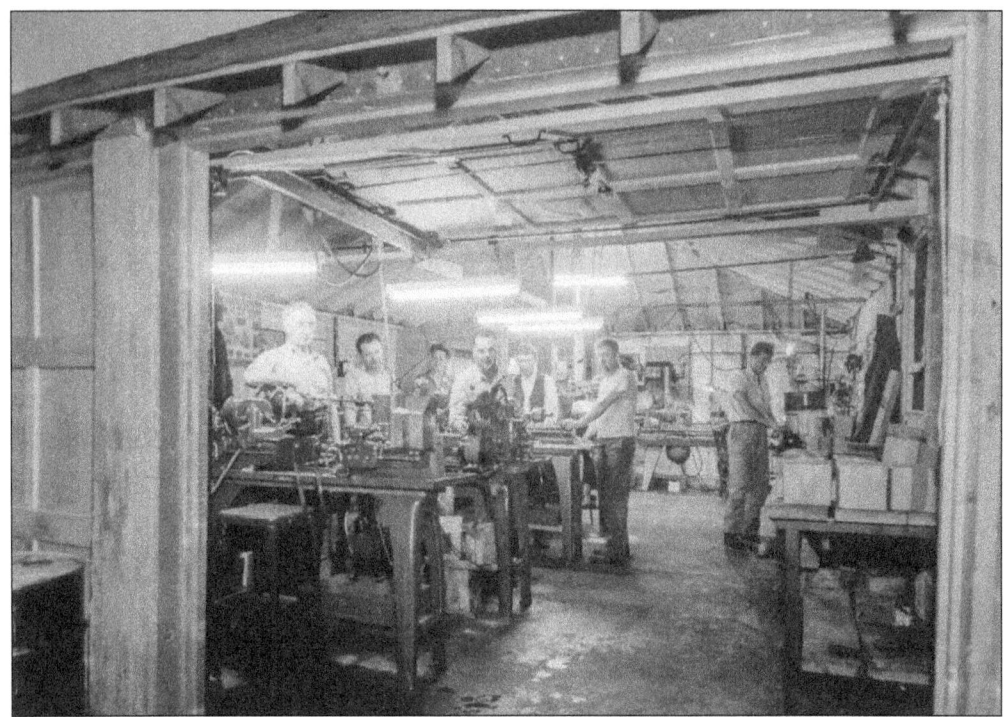

Similar to many high school vocational programs, trade shops were a predominantly male environment at the facilities. Metal and automotive shops were a favorite for many mechanically inclined individuals. Above, at Central Islip State Hospital, a view of the metal lathe area is seen in the 1960s. Here, parts were machined for countless uses around the hospital, from car parts to door hardware. Below, two men are working in the metal shop with a stick welder. From this photograph, it would be difficult to guess they were on the grounds of a state hospital. Work activity allowed for a normalization level that helped prepare patients for careers outside of the hospital.

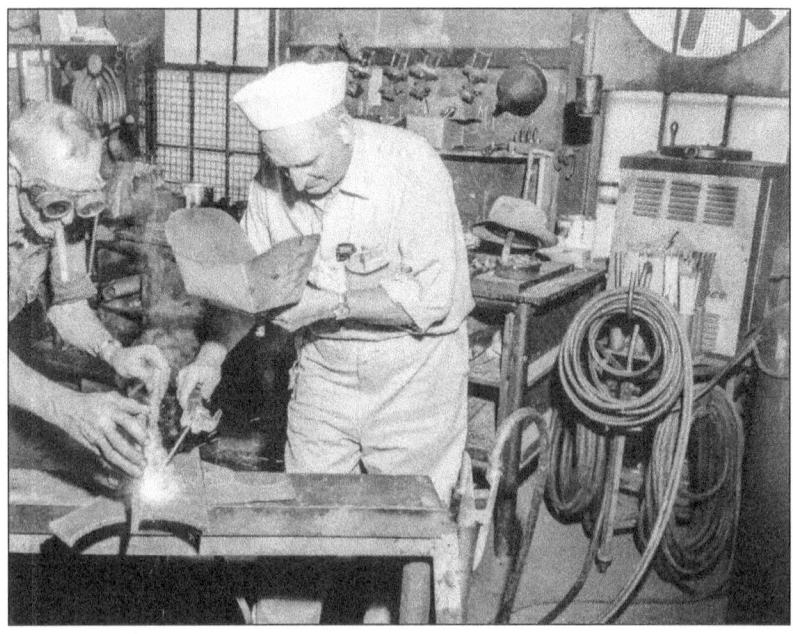

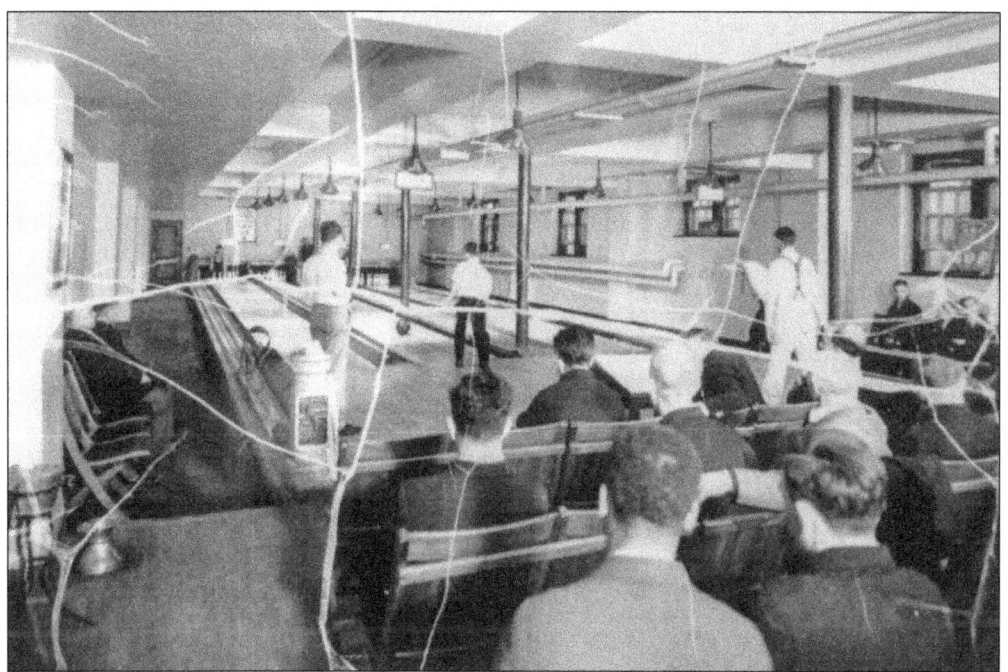

Bowling was a popular recreational activity at the institutions long before the advent of electricity. At one point, there was a state hospital bowling league where patients would compete against other state facilities. Above, a manual bowling alley at Central Islip State Hospital is pictured in the early 1920s. The man at the end of the lane would reset the pins and toss the ball down a wooden ball return. Below, a group of men at Kings Park State Hospital pose for a team photograph in the 1950s in the "White House." The White House was a wooden cottage on the grounds used for recreation.

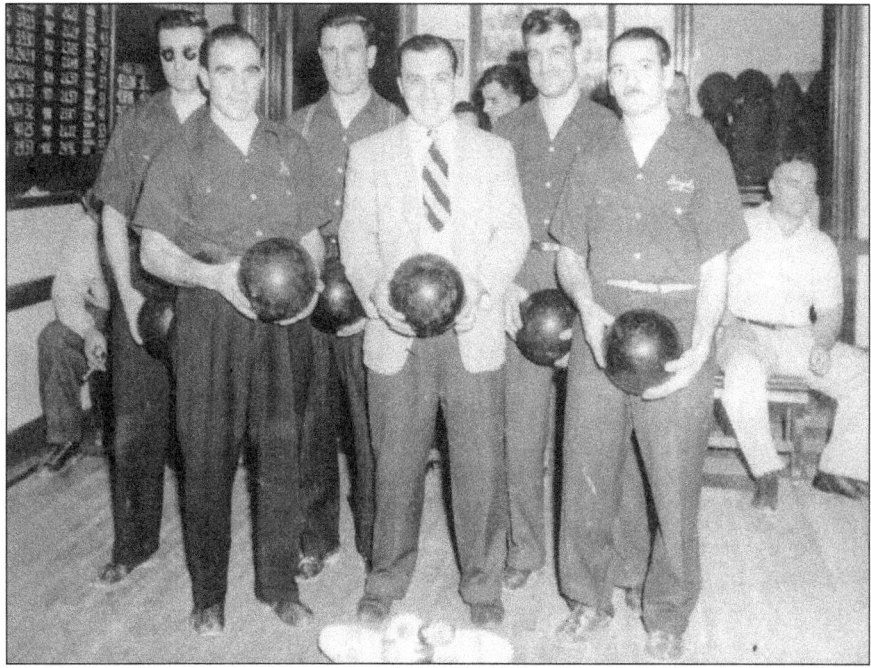

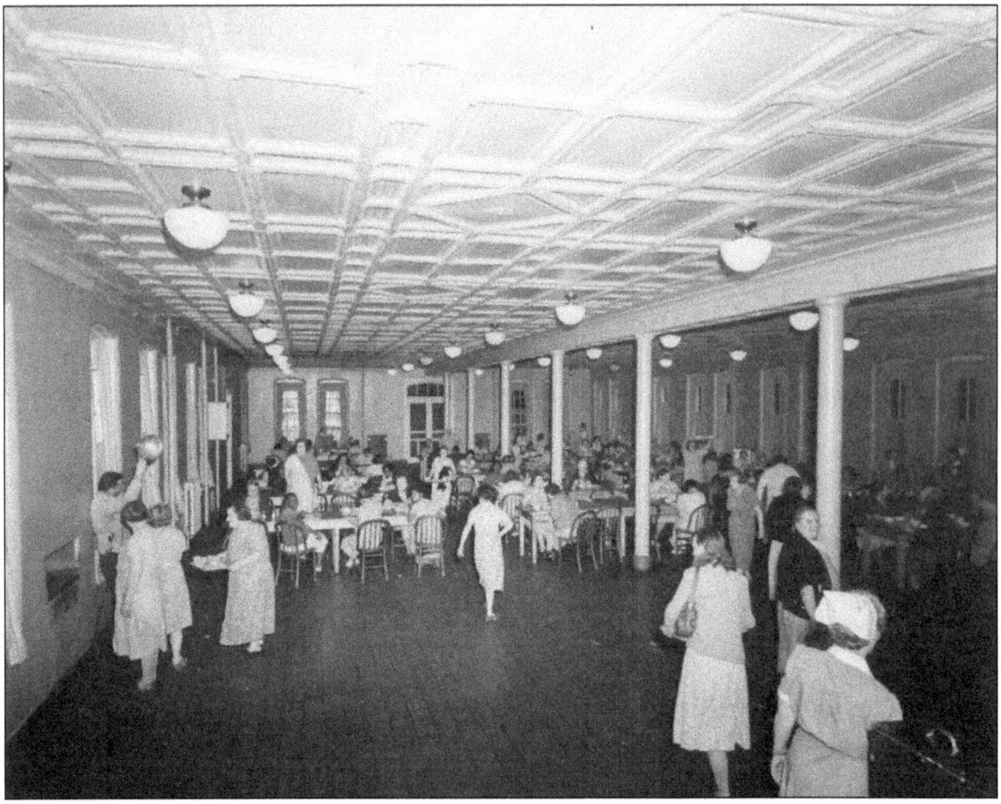

Meals were a time when everyone in a ward had an opportunity to socialize together. Many meals were served in massive dining halls, similar to ones found at a college. This is a look at Central Islip State Hospital in the 1950s during peak operations. With 9,000-plus patients, each consuming three meals a day, the kitchen staff were very busy.

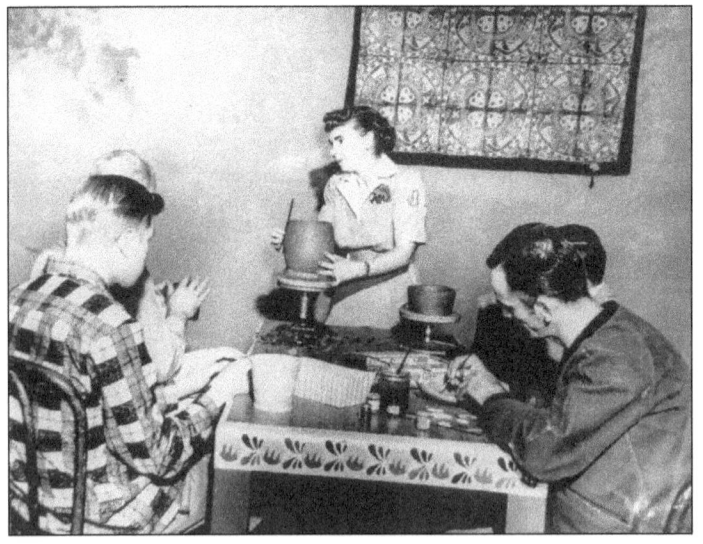

Many different recreational and occupational opportunities were offered to patients. Once one mastered a skill, they would typically move on to another group of skills. Here, at Pilgrim State Hospital in the 1940s, a small group of men work on ceramic painting. An occupational therapy aide works on small turntables to craft ceramic pots.

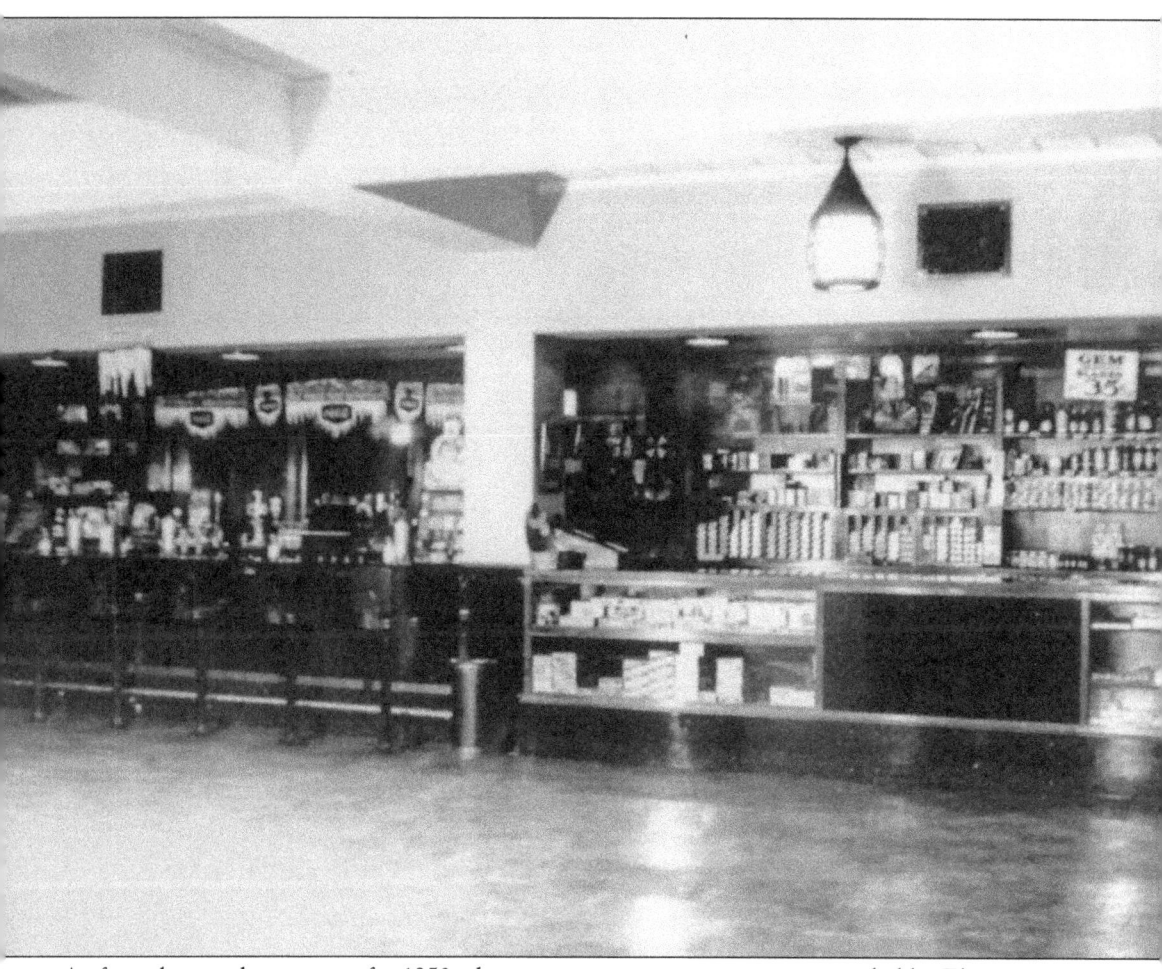

At first glance, this image of a 1950s drugstore counter may seem unremarkable. This store, however, had great meaning to the patients at the hospital. The community, or "token," store at Central Islip State Hospital was a link to the many comforts of home. Patients who worked earned a wage paid in tokens, which were paper cards marked with the financial amounts they equated to. It was essentially the currency of the hospital. Token economy, as it is known, was utilized around the country for decades to reinforce prosocial behavior through positive rewards. To the left sits a counter where milkshakes and fountain soda could be purchased. On the right, cigarettes, hard candy, and sundries were available. The token system was long successful in the rehabilitation of many patients who previously were unable to perform tasks or participate in social groups prior to admission.

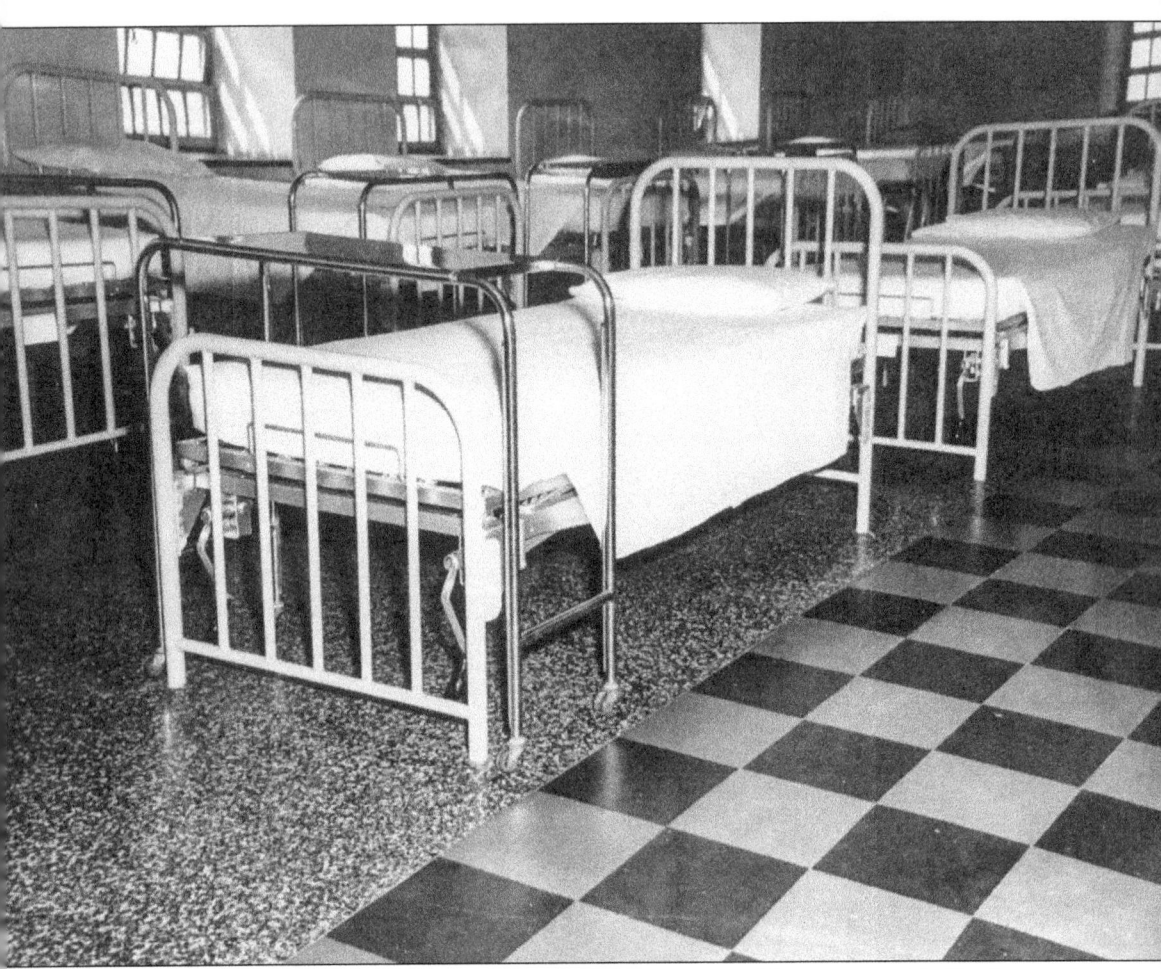

In the living units, having a clean and tidy ward was an essential function provided by the nursing staff, often with help from the patients. Staff took great pride in the condition of their wards. Informal competitions among the staff over who had cleaner units remains common in behavioral healthcare. In this photograph at Kings Park State Hospital in Building 93, crisply folded hospital corners are evident on the beds. Each pillowcase is precisely placed with the opening side facing away from the door. The floor is polished and waxed to a high gloss. A critical element of life at the institution was dedication to the welfare of the patients, down to the smallest details.

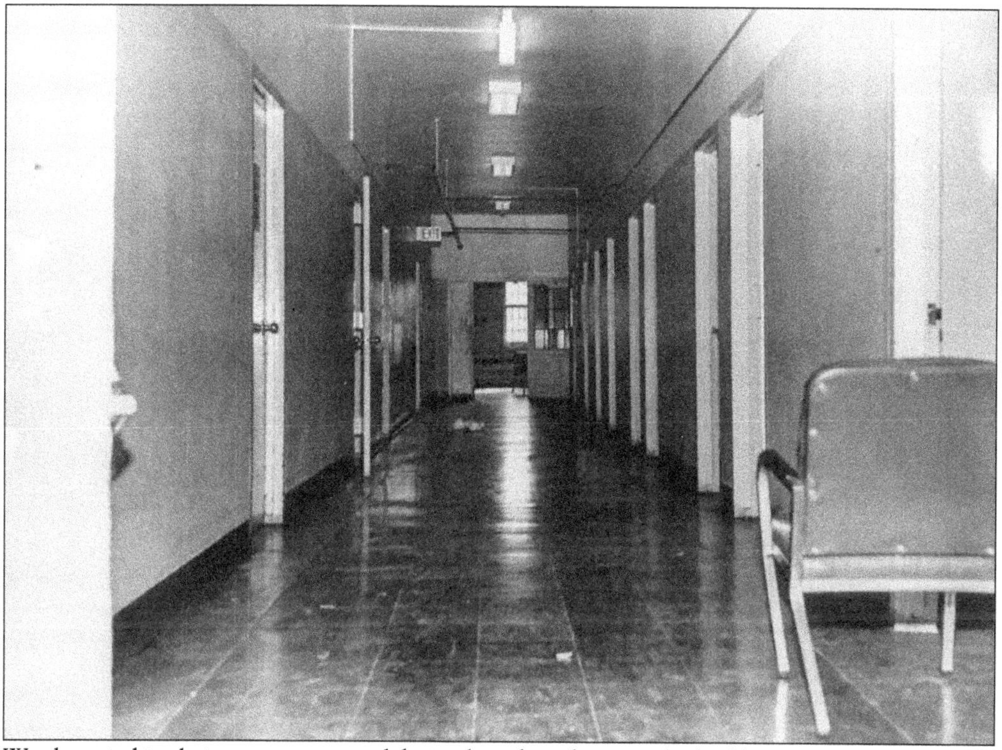

Wards varied in their appearance and design based on the time the building was constructed and its use. This unit inside Central Islip State Hospital's Building 7 is seen looking from the dormitory all the way to the day hall beyond the open door in the background. This building served as an admission unit for many years and was one of the last to close in 1996.

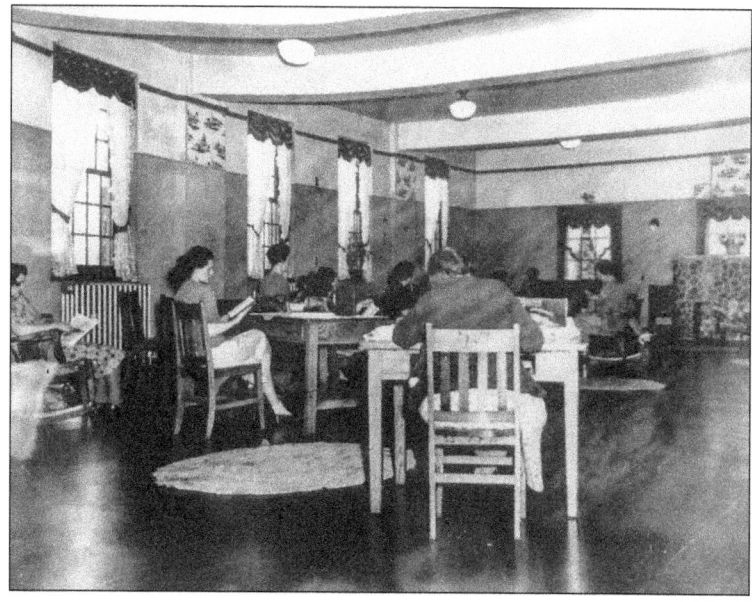

Seen here is a female day hall inside Central Islip State Hospital's Building 7. This was an admissions unit for women in the 1960s, when this photograph was taken. Admissions was the first place a patient would be brought upon arrival to the hospital. After an observation period, patients were placed in the building most conducive for their recovery.

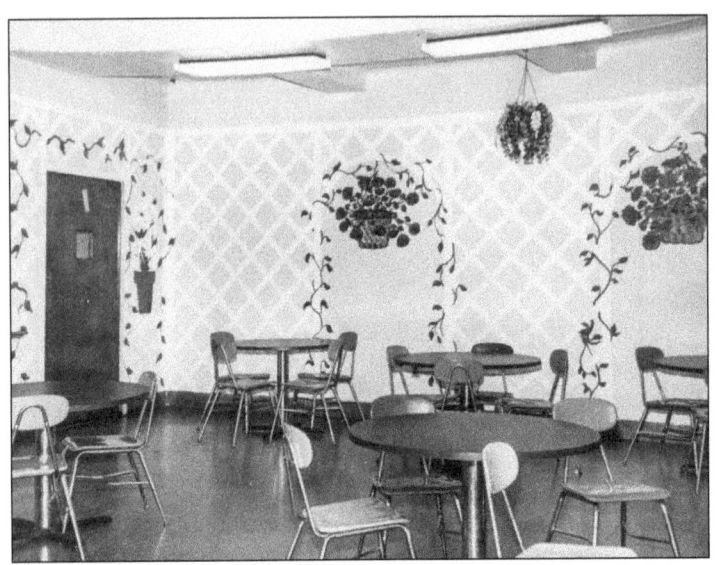

Often, if a space could be made more visually stimulating though paint or decoration, it became a project for a patient who was interested. Here, a once-ordinary dining room in Building 7 at Central Islip State Hospital is painted to resemble an outdoor terrace, with plants suspended from the ceiling. Simple projects like these cost almost nothing and provided big changes to rooms once sterile in appearance.

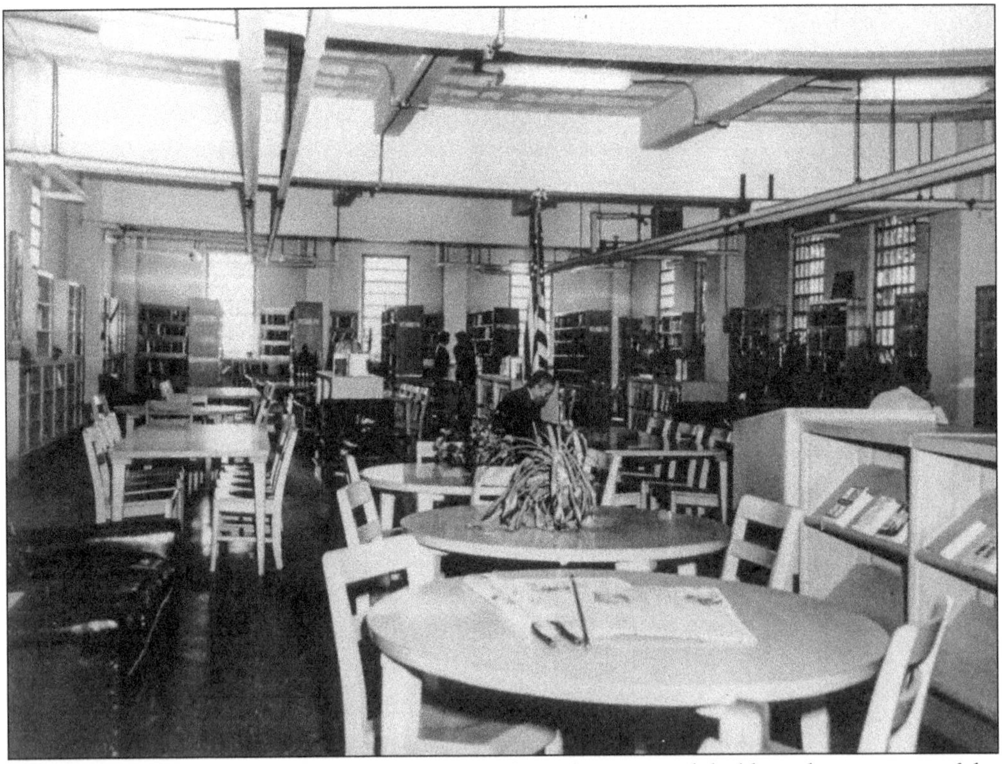

The patient library was a popular destination. Before television took hold, reading was one of the few places to turn for information and entertainment. Many patients were avid readers and were permitted to take books back to their wards with them. The library in Building 127 at Central Islip State Hospital is seen here in the 1950s.

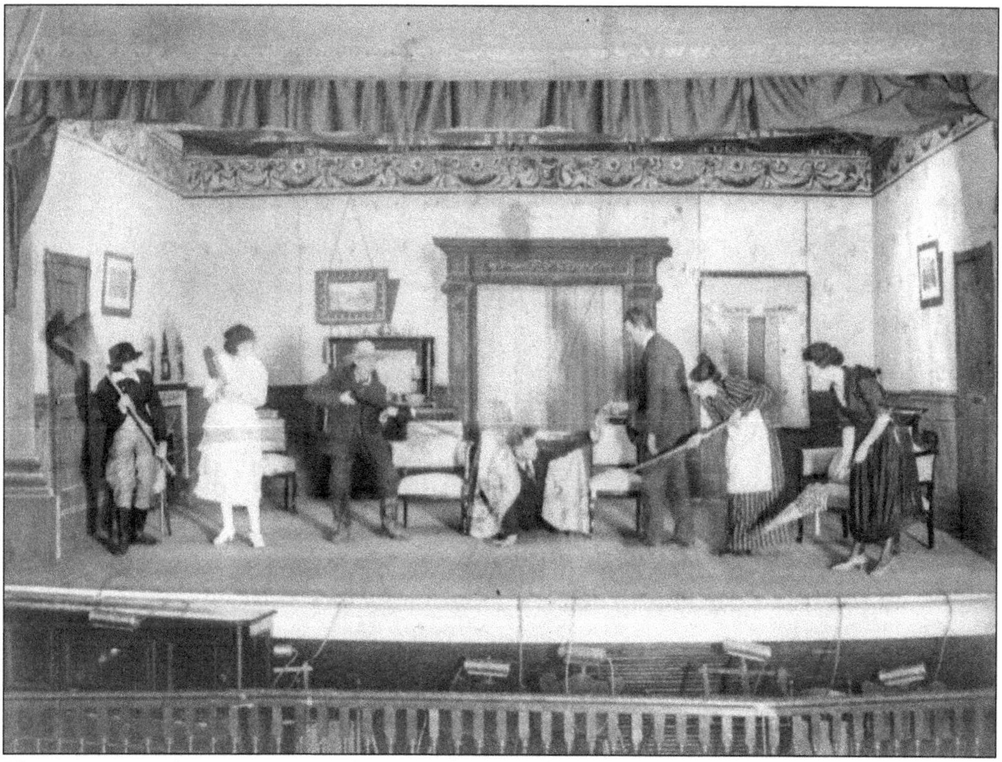

Plays were a regular occurrence at Kings Park State Hospital. This particular production captured on a glass plate in the 1910s took place in the wooden recreation building that was replaced by York Hall. Note the player piano and orchestra pit in the foreground. Shows were an opportunity for many talented patients to feel accomplished, while also providing entertainment for their peers. (Courtesy of the Kings Park Heritage Museum.)

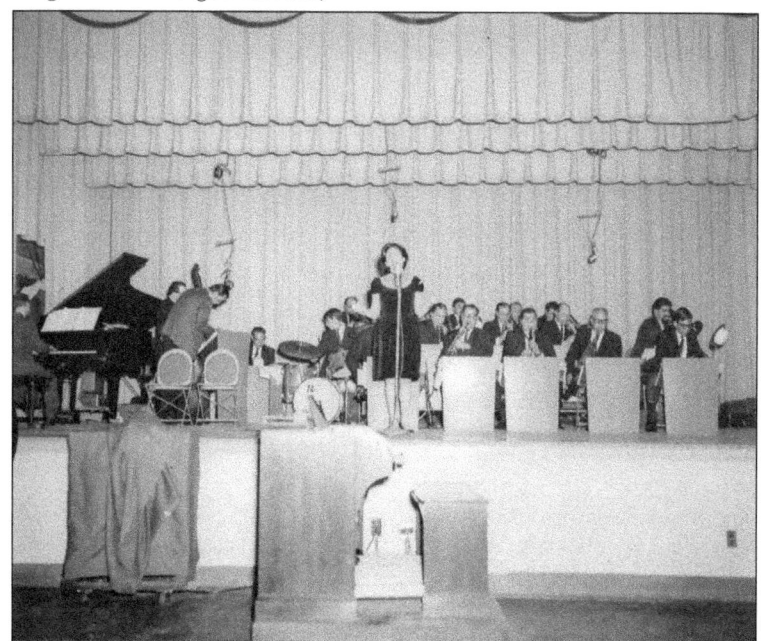

An evening jazz performance at Pilgrim State Hospital in the 1960s is captured on film in Building 26, the assembly hall. To the right, members of the band play woodwind instruments. In the center, a woman sings. It was not uncommon for entertainers to volunteer their time to perform for the patients at the hospital free of charge.

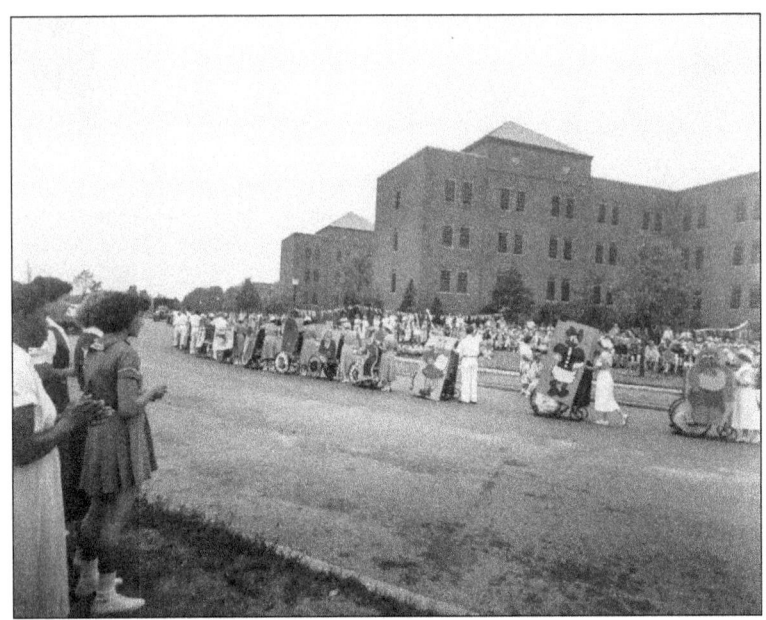

Parades were a hospital-wide event that stopped the ordinary business of the facility at least once a year. Ways to include the patients who were less physically capable were frequently a consideration. Here, at Central Islip State Hospital, wheelchair-bound individuals are participating in the parade.

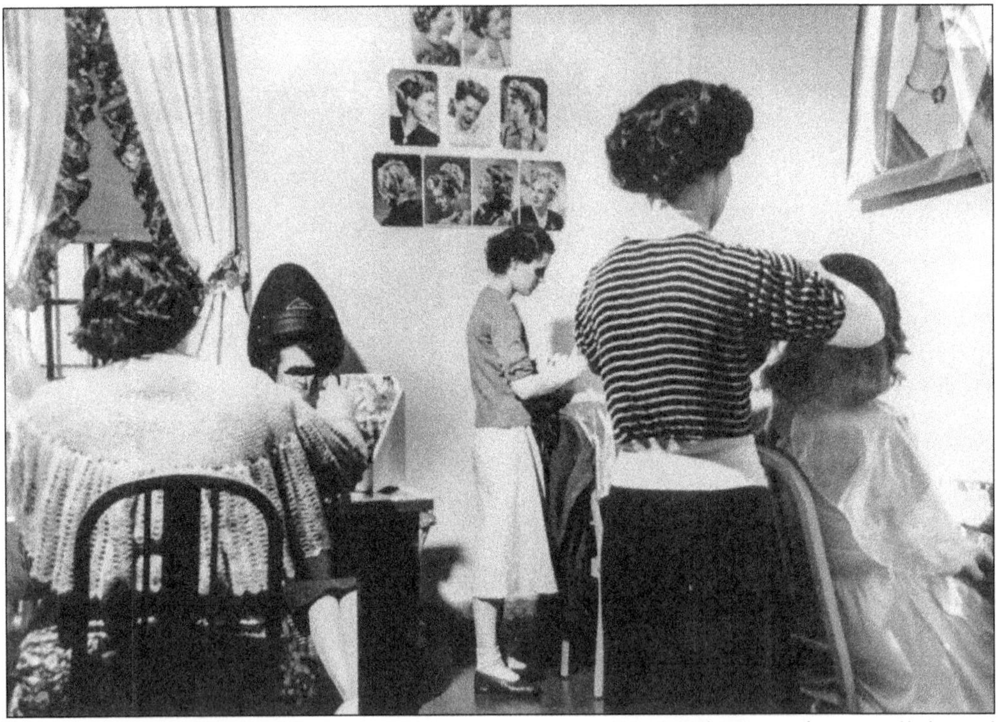

Grooming greatly affects the way people feel about themselves. When people are well dressed and comb their hair, they often feel more positive. In light of this, making sure women had the opportunity to visit a beautician while hospitalized was thought a necessity. Here, a group of female patients visit the beauticians at Pilgrim State Hospital.

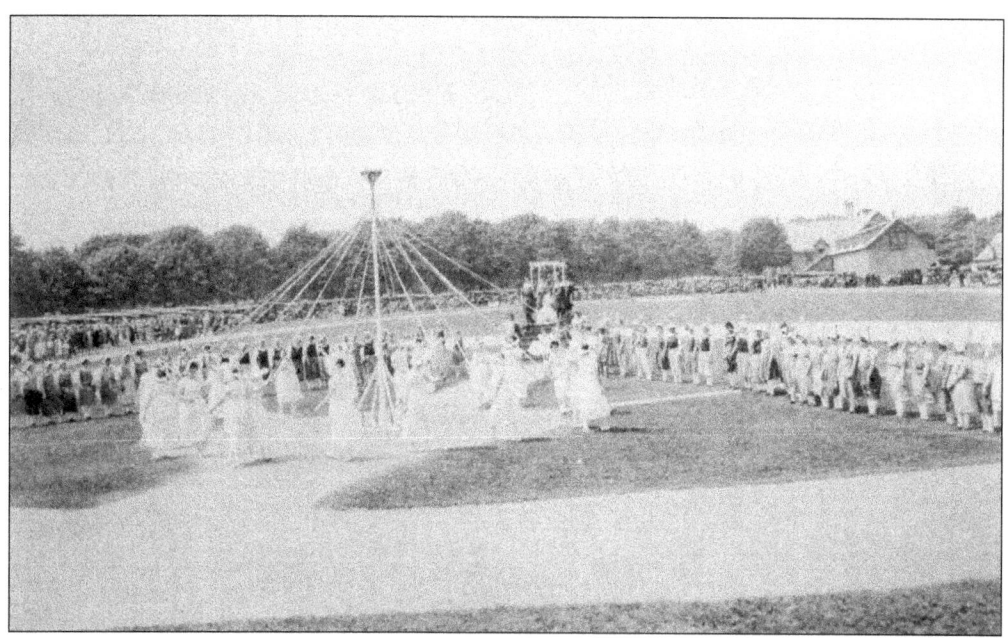

Outdoor celebrations were a signal for those living at the state hospitals that spring had arrived. Patients enjoyed the park-like grounds and took time to socialize with people they normally did not get to see because of the size of the facilities. Above and below, women can be seen taking part in a Maypole celebration at Central Islip State Hospital in the 1920s. As the name would suggest, traditionally, Maypole celebrations were held on May 1. A tall pole was erected on the baseball diamond, with colorful cloth strands that were wound around the pole as part of a dance.

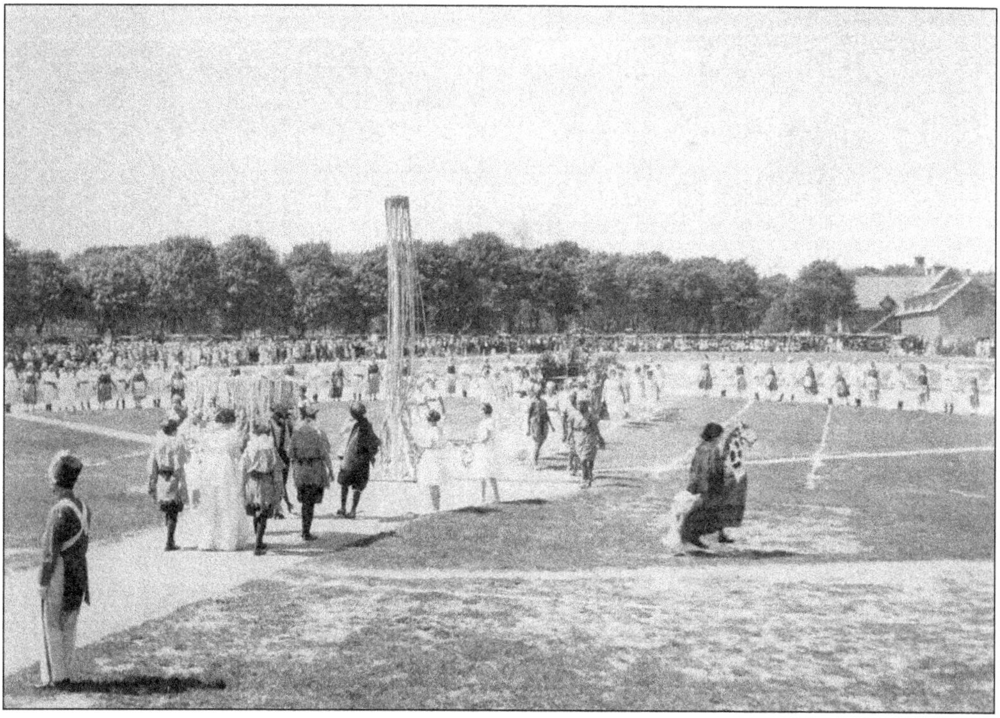

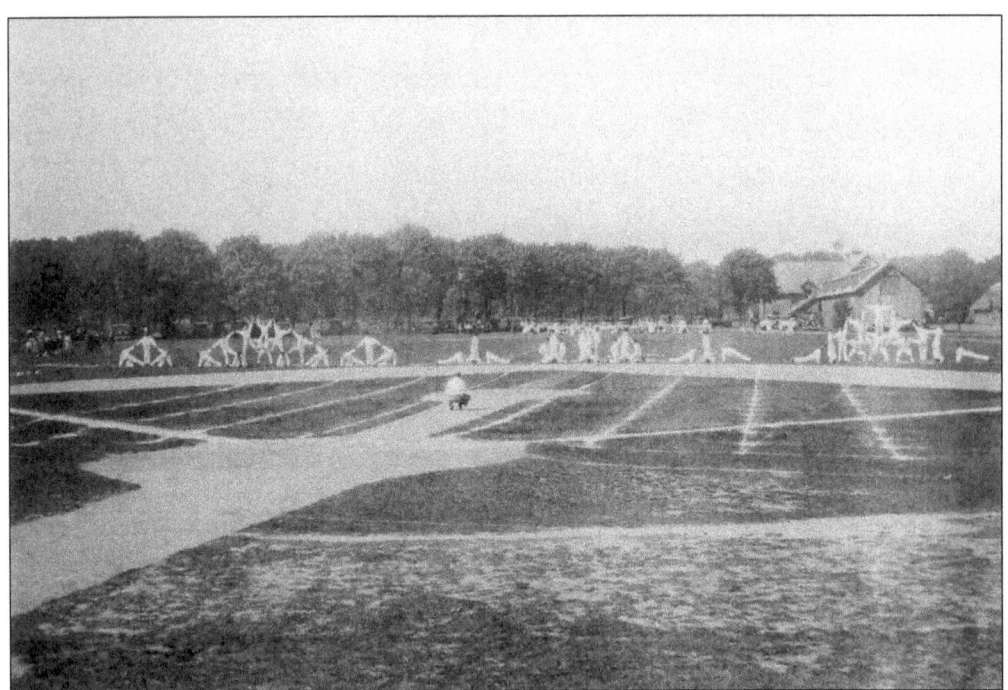

Physical activity was highly regarded and greatly increased under Dr. Smith at Central Islip State Hospital. Dr. Smith believed sitting idly did not contribute to the general well-being of patients. He published several volumes on treatment improvements in public institutions. Cooperative activities to accomplish gymnastic-like formations involved a high degree of cognitive activation and socialization among peers. In these images from the 1920s, pyramid exercises with men can be seen outside on a spring day. Not only was this type of recreation a benefit to those engaged, but it also provided entertainment for spectators.

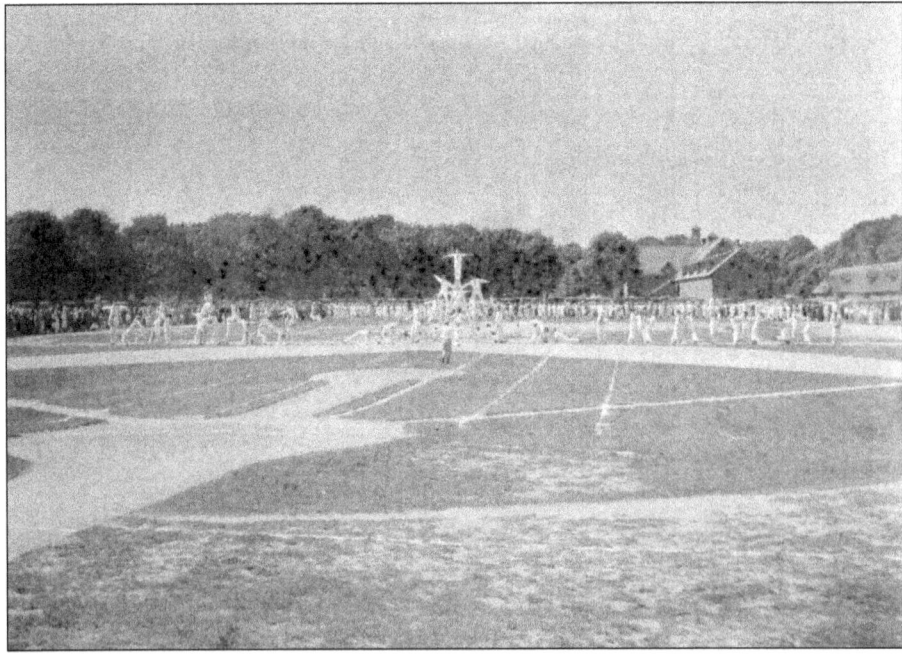

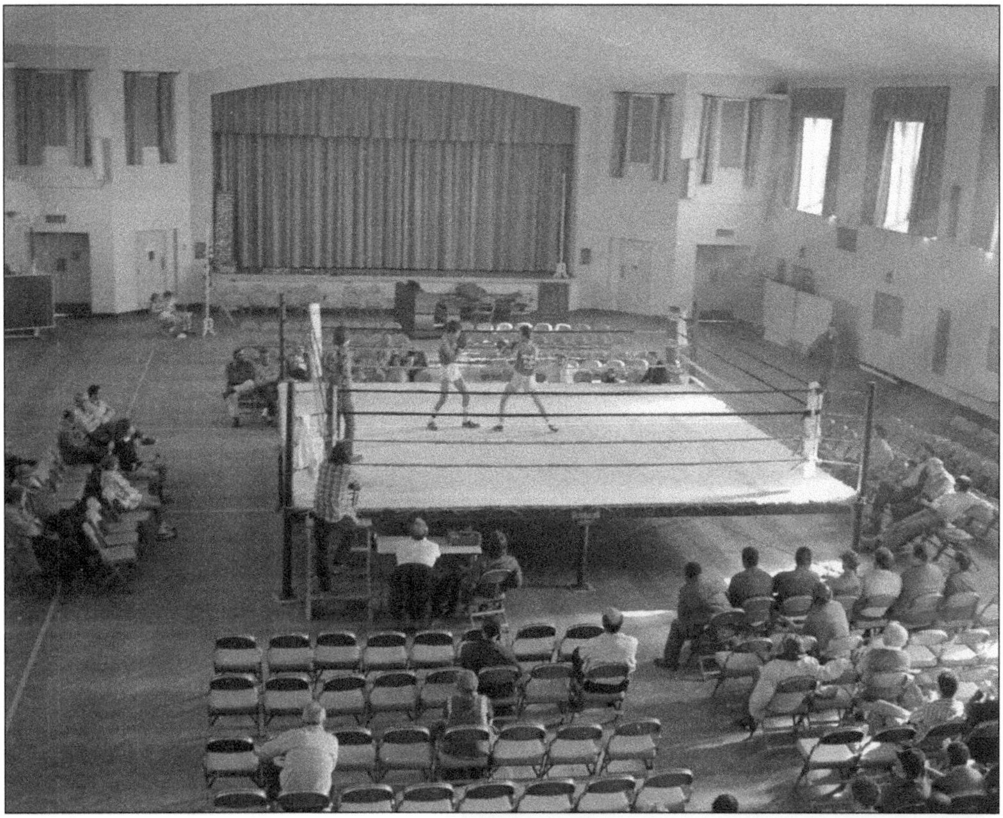

Over the years, many athletes and entertainers visited the state hospitals to perform for the patients and staff. In this 1960s photograph taken at Pilgrim State Hospital, boxers put on a fight for spectators inside the assembly hall. Entertainment like this would often be charity work done by the performers at little to no cost to the hospital.

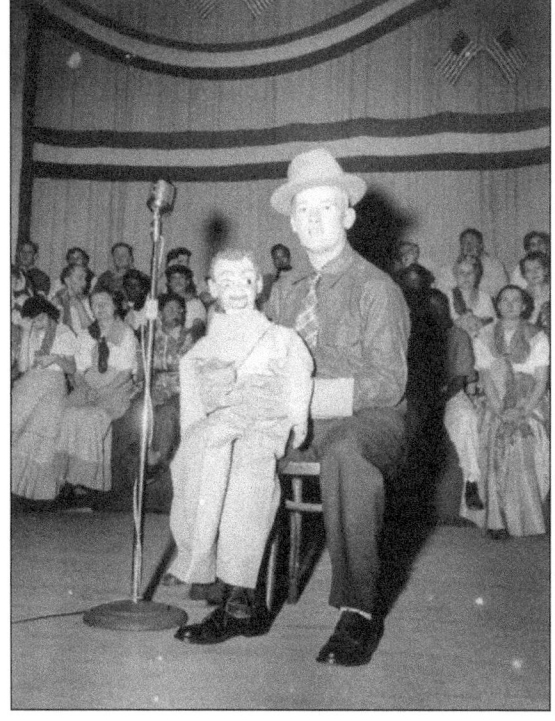

Other entertainers included staff and patients who possessed talents in the performing arts. This evening comedy show was held at Pilgrim State Hospital in the 1960s. A man and his ventriloquist doll act out a skit for audience members gathered in the assembly hall. Humor was a common denominator for many of the skits put on at the hospitals, as laughter has many positive therapeutic qualities.

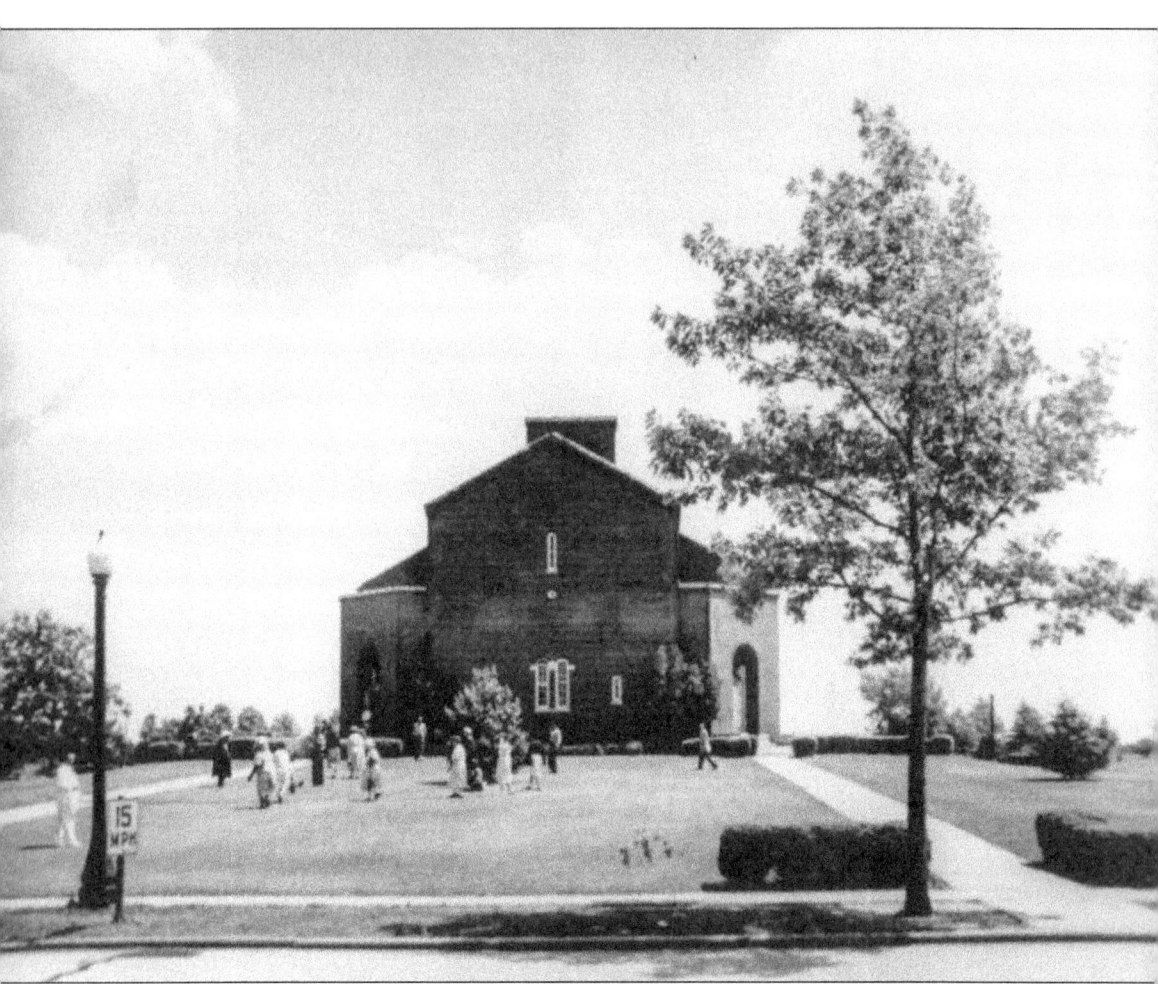

Building 26 at Pilgrim State Hospital was built shortly after the campus opened in 1931. Constructed for the purpose of entertainment, it was a building of great significance to everyone who lived or worked on grounds. On the ground floor, a stage and portable seating allowed for large numbers of individuals to assemble for business or leisure. The same area was also used as the basketball and indoor sports court in addition to being the space where social events and dances were put on. In the old days of the hospital, it was the only place men and women were permitted to socialize. The community store and bowling alley were in the basement. Providing recreation and physical activity to patients allowed a firm foundation to begin addressing the emotional problems that brought them to the facility. Ensuring basic needs were met before addressing complex issues was a successful treatment for many decades.

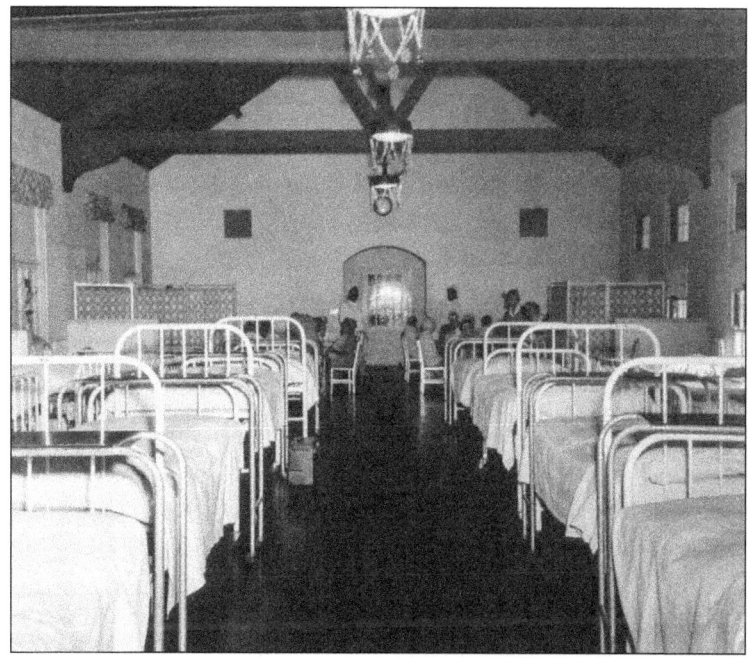

The A and B Group at Central Islip State Hospital is seen here in the 1950s. When this photograph was taken, the hospital was at high capacity, causing some wards to be crowded. This geriatric unit dormitory is quite full, with just a few inches between beds. In the background, nurses are conducting a therapy group.

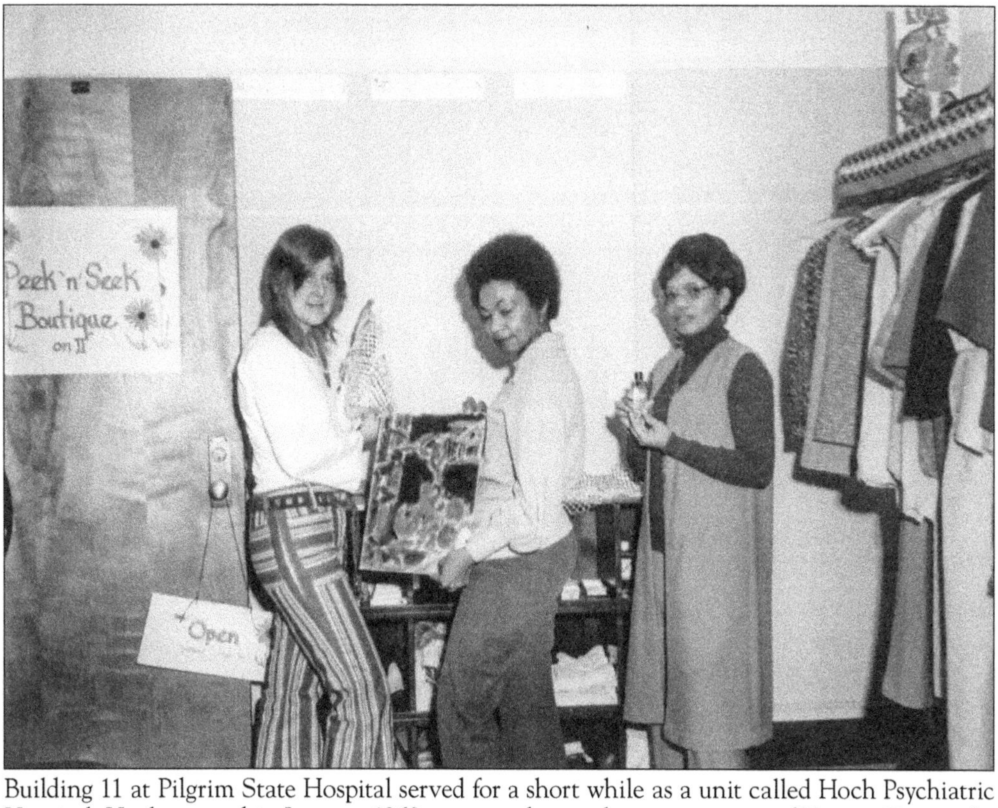

Building 11 at Pilgrim State Hospital served for a short while as a unit called Hoch Psychiatric Hospital. Hoch opened in January 1969 to serve the southeastern region of Nassau County for adults 19 and over. Hoch was small and averaged about 95 patients per day in the 1970s. Seen here, the women's boutique at Hoch provided goods for female patients at the facility.

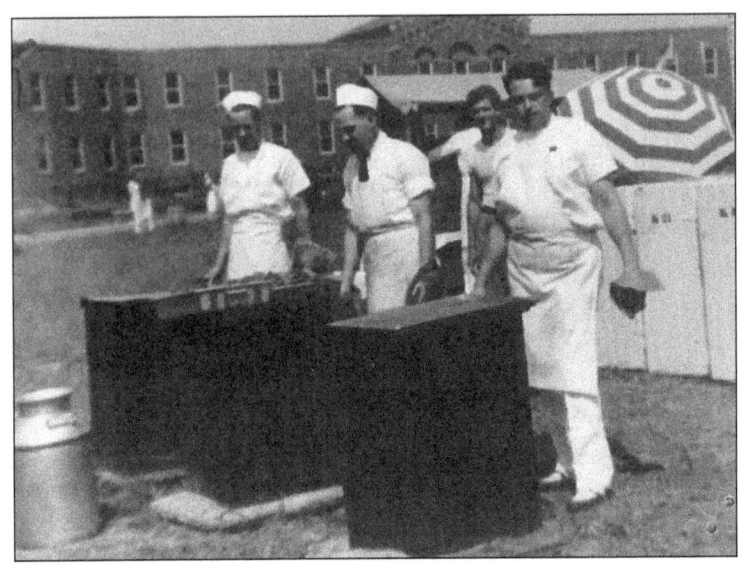

Summertime at Pilgrim State Hospital meant many activities on the enormous lawns of the campus. Picnics were held routinely for buildings or different program groups. Here, in the 1960s, some of the kitchen staff are serving up a hot dog lunch one summer day in the center of the campus known as "the Nurses Circle."

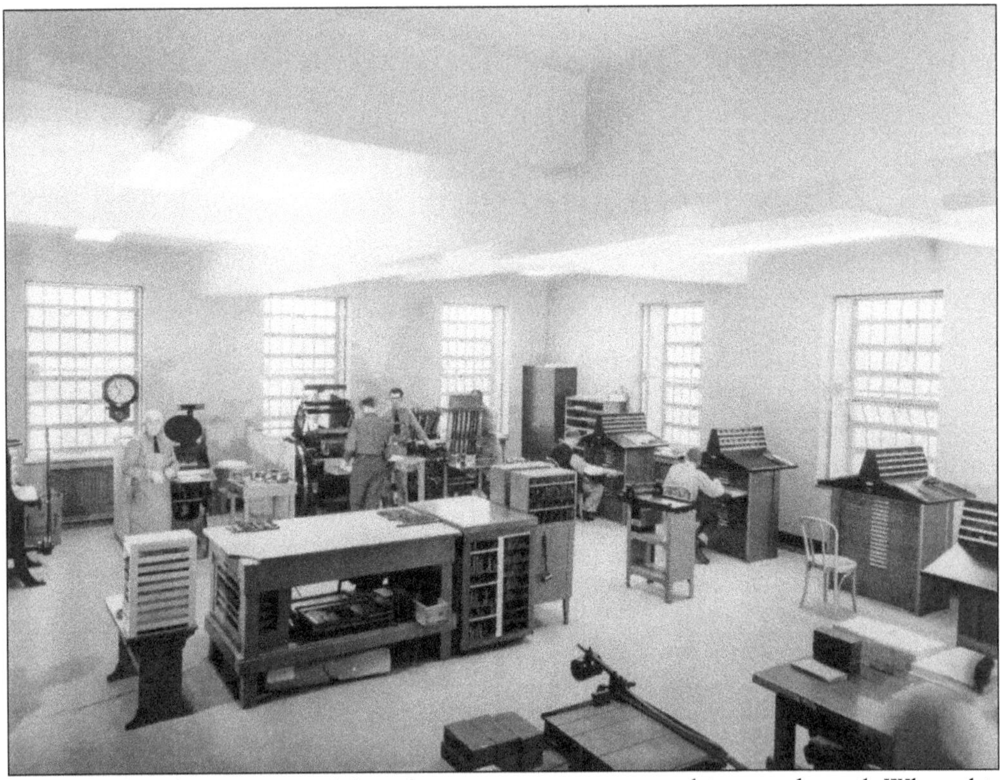

It is difficult today to imagine life without computers, copy machines, and email. When this photograph was taken in the Corcoran Complex at Central Islip State Hospital in the 1950s, the print shop was the heart of communication for the hospital. Forms, greeting cards, newspapers, and virtually all printed materials were crafted here. Men work on setting up blocks to print forms with an ink press.

Close inspection of the canvas reveals that this man was a talented artist. A wonderful surprise for many of the activities staff was to discover the often hidden talents patients possessed. It was a sobering reminder for many that all patients who came through the doors had lives of varying circumstances and experience despite their present mental state.

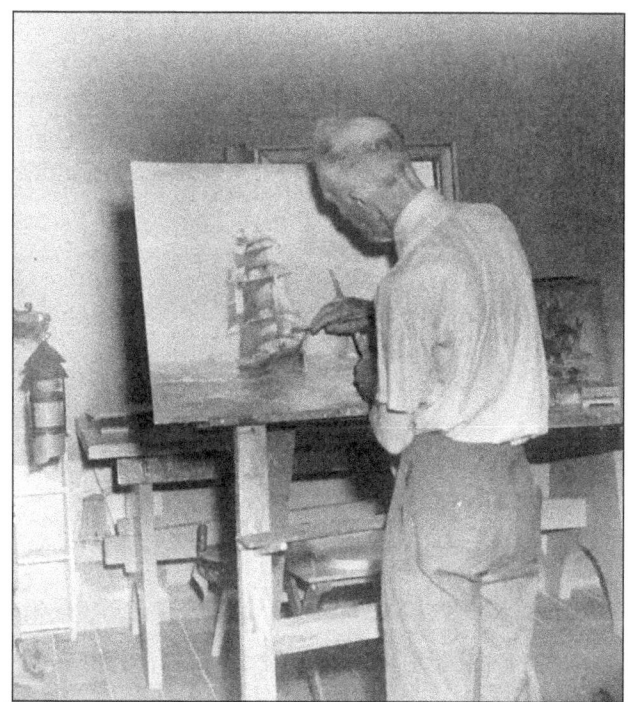

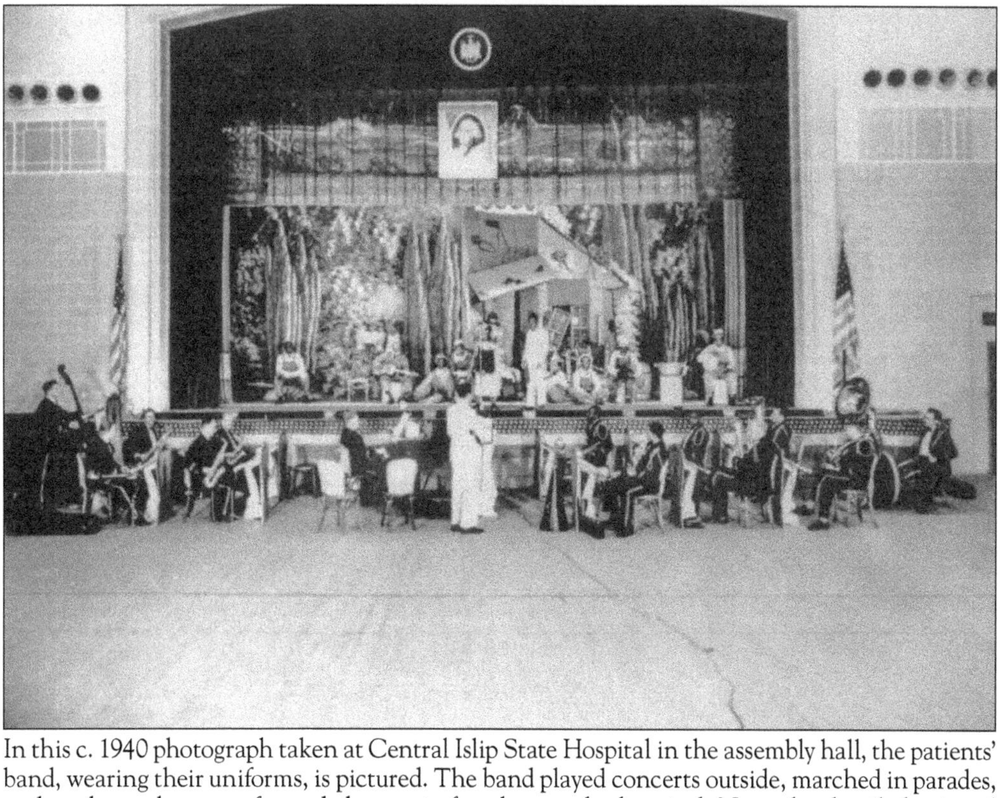

In this c. 1940 photograph taken at Central Islip State Hospital in the assembly hall, the patients' band, wearing their uniforms, is pictured. The band played concerts outside, marched in parades, and as shown here, performed the music for plays at the hospital. Note the detailed painted backdrop on the stage.

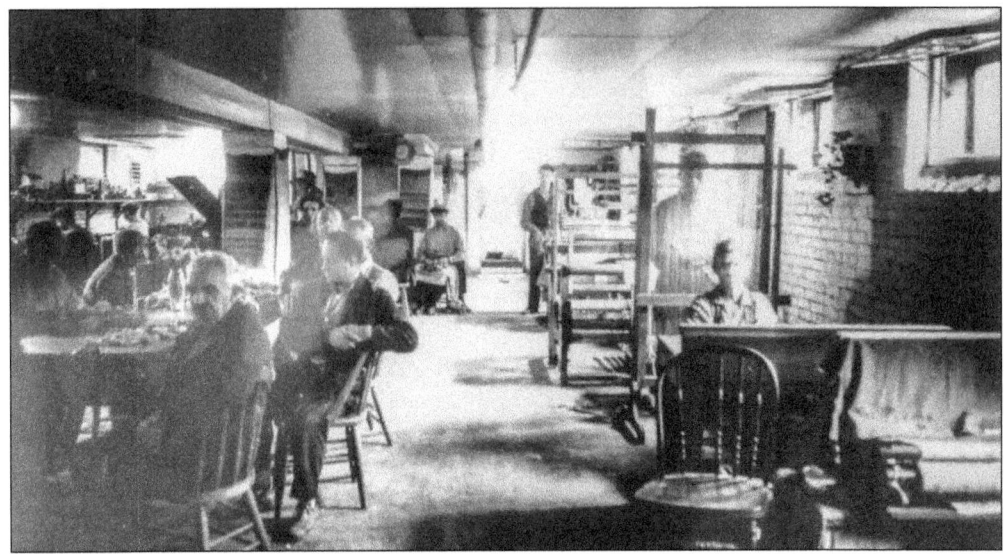

Before the construction of buildings dedicated to activities, shops were located wherever space permitted. Here, at Kings Park State Hospital, a male weaving class is located in the basement of Group I. Space on living units was needed for lodging and clinical needs. As a result, basements became the norm for recreation space. (Courtesy of the Kings Park Heritage Museum.)

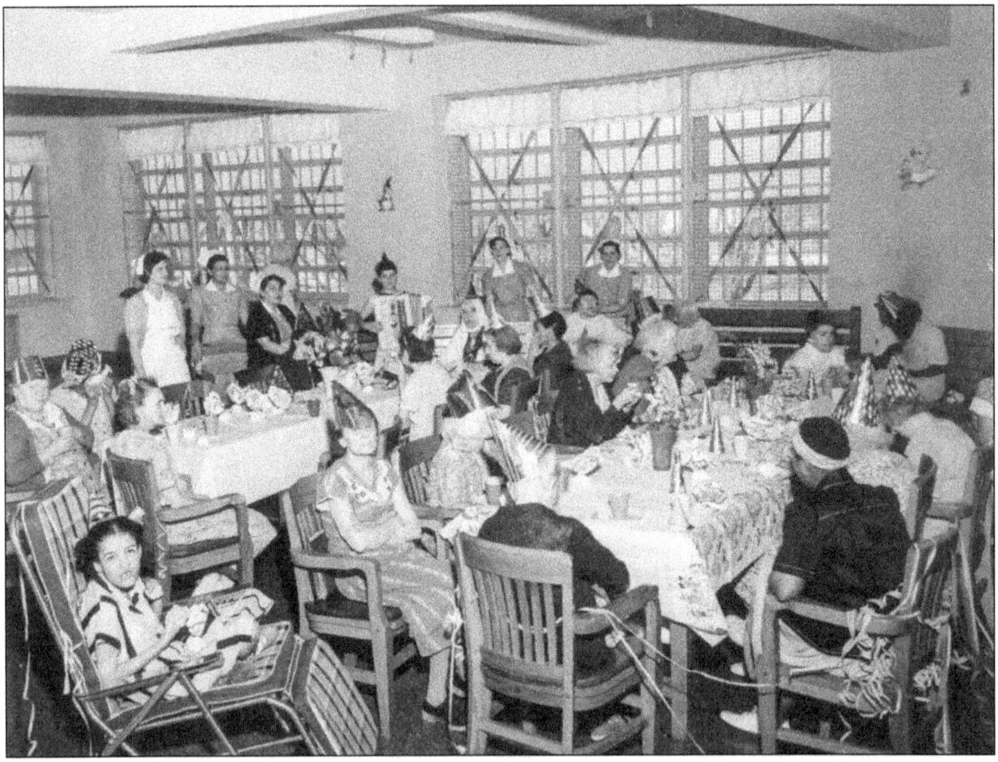

Many patients who lived at the state hospitals had few or no visitors. The staff and fellow patients became in their own way a pseudo-family. Holidays were celebrated in groups so patients could be included and not brood alone. Here at Central Islip State Hospital in the 1950s, a Passover meal is celebrated family style in Corcoran Building.

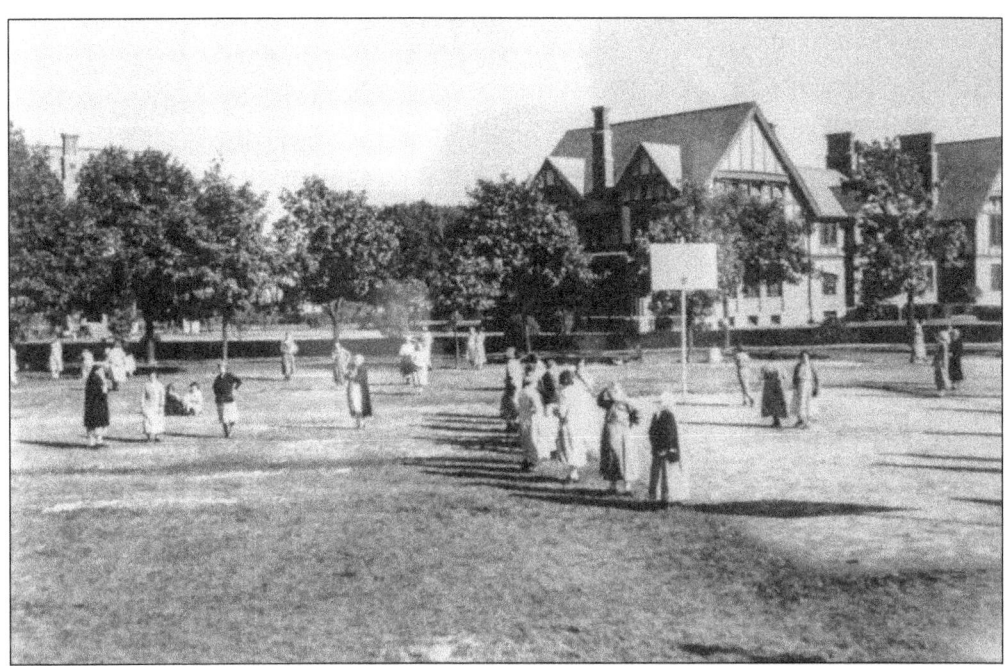

Central Islip State Hospital was the most distinguished of the Long Island state hospitals in terms of physical fitness. It was largely the result of Supt. Dr. Smith, who was an advocate and pioneer in assisting recreational therapy. In 1932, Smith's work was acknowledged in a short book, *Physical Training & Recreation in a Mental Hospital*. Patients were separated by levels of cognitive function in order to assign the intensity and difficulty of cooperative movement to be performed. Dance and music were paired with activities. Today, music and dance are well respected as recreation therapy–based interventions. Below, a formation of women engage in one such session in the 1930s. Above, leisure time is held on the grounds adjacent to the Smith Group at Central Islip.

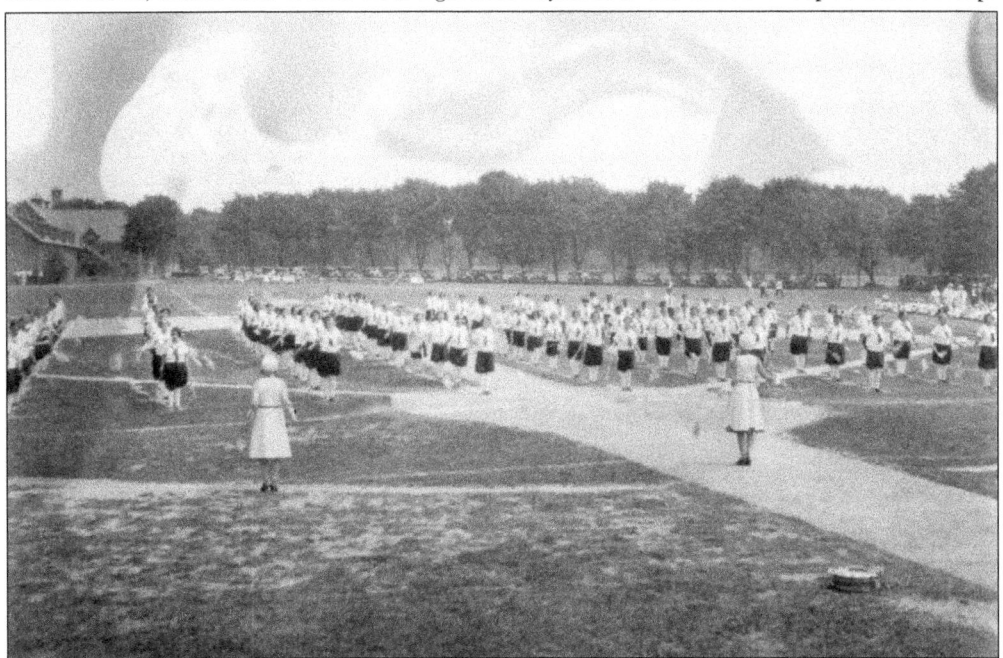

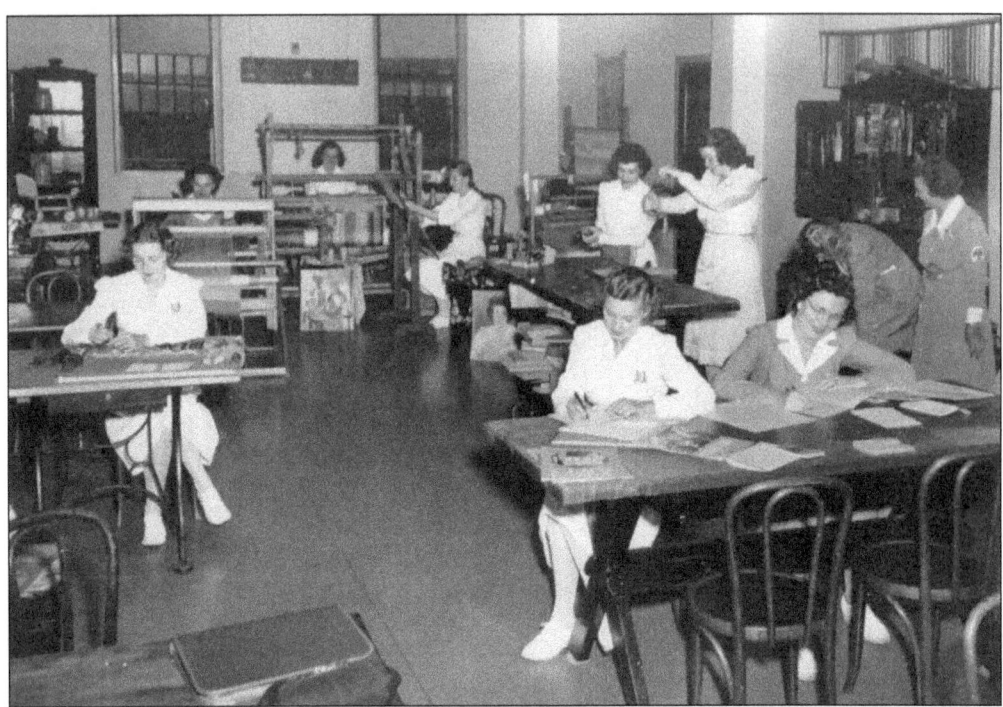

In order to teach patients different occupational or recreational activities, therapy staff would get together and share techniques. Above, at Pilgrim State Hospital, female therapy staff (wearing darker uniforms) teach student nurses (white uniforms) craft activities. Although nurses mainly provided medical care, an understanding of how each department operated in the facility was a part of the students' training. Below, a man works on a quilt in an activities building around the 1940s. The imprinting on the cloth was done with linoleum blocks. A block of linoleum was carved into a design to be used as a pattern stamp.

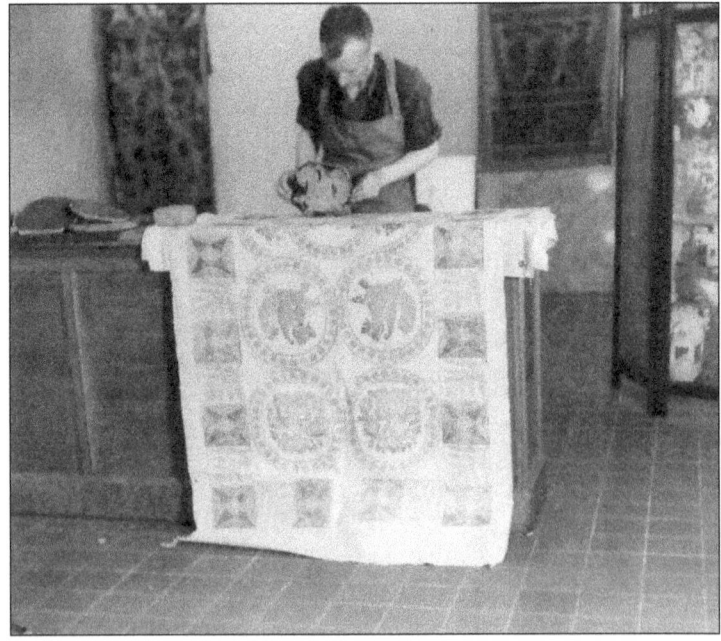

A woman works with scraps of wool and burlap to craft a rug. Rug hooking, as it is known, originated in England in the 19th century, where factory workers would gather scraps of fabrics from leftover mill material. Similarly, scraps of textile from other projects at the hospital were reclaimed and used in ornamental pieces.

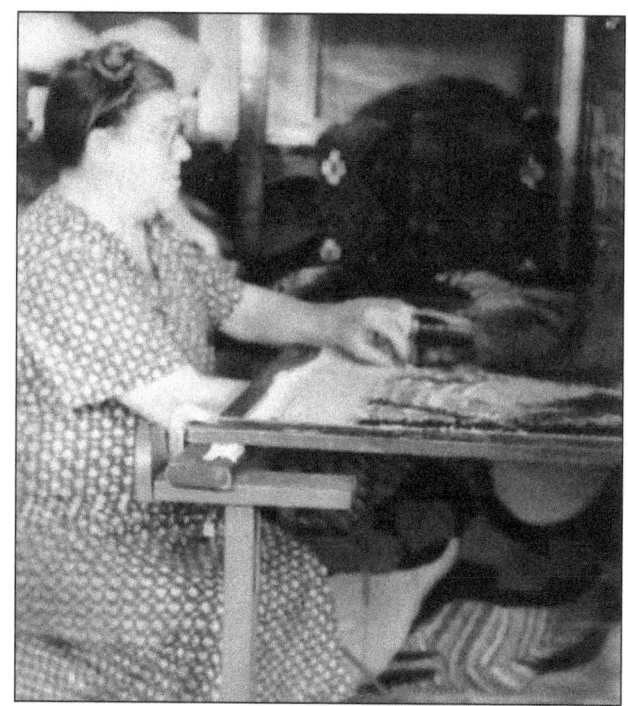

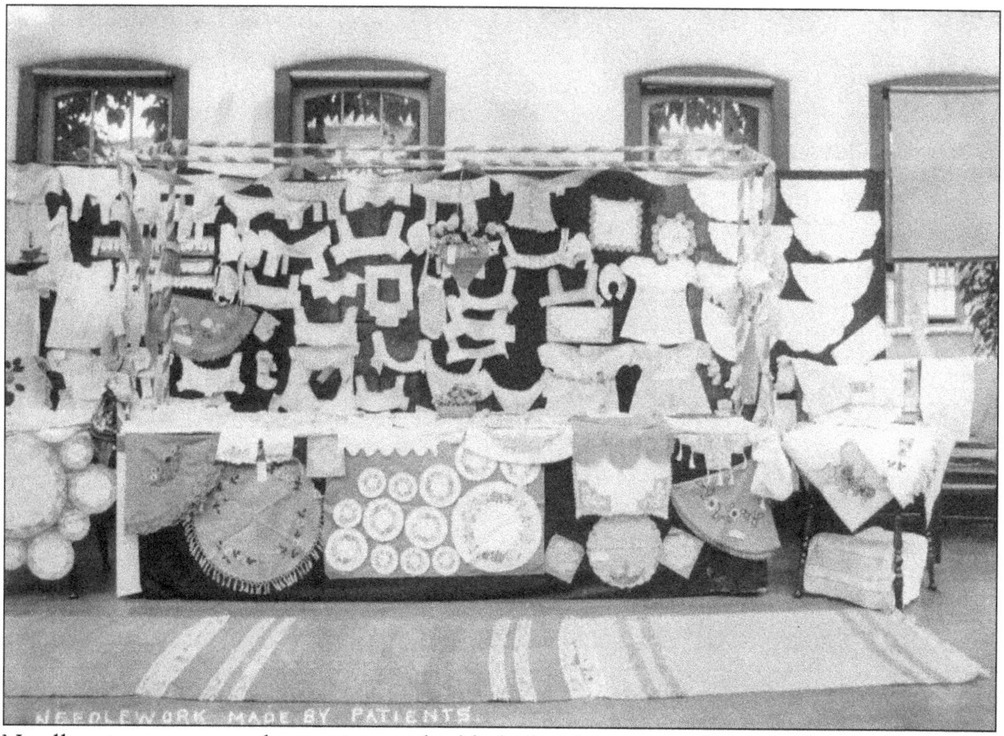

Needlepoint was a popular pastime with elderly female patients. It required virtually costless thread and small cloth swatches. Patients would often congregate and sew in a circle in a dayroom, discussing the happenings at the hospital. An occupational therapy display of needlepoint in the 1920s at Kings Park State Hospital is seen here.

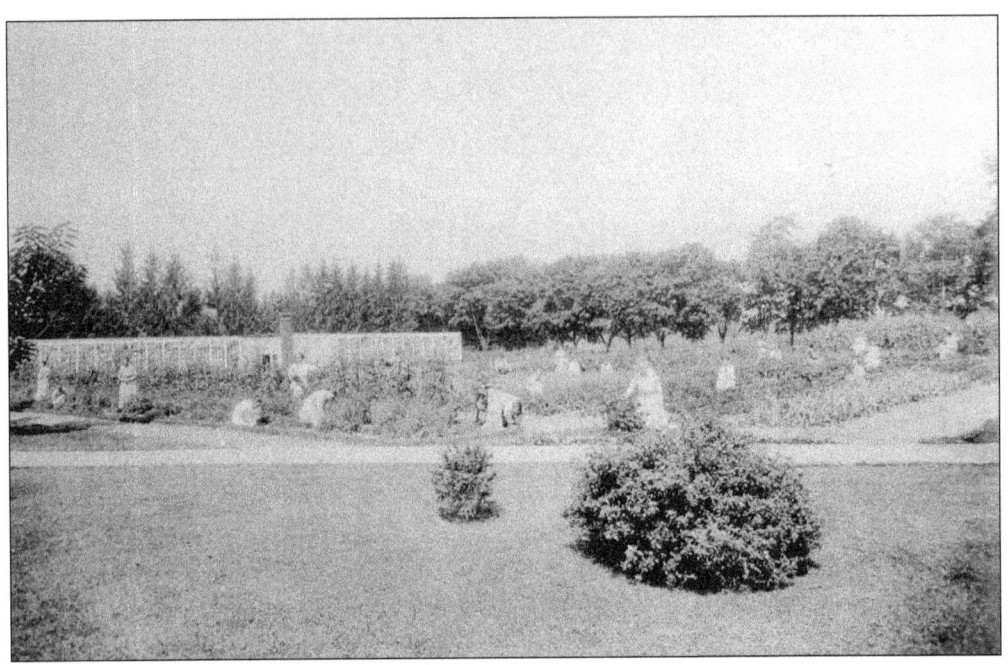

Horticulture was interwoven into many facets of life at the institutions. Ornamental gardening was one way of maintaining a serene atmosphere while providing purposeful activity. Each building was supplied with a garden space for its use. In both of these images at Central Islip State Hospital in the 1940s, women tend to a field of flowers. Above, a hothouse can be seen in the background. Here, seeds were germinated into plants ready for use on the grounds. Below, women don straw hats to provide sun protection on a summer day while picking wild raspberries. To the right, an arch-shaped trellis appears to be in bloom.

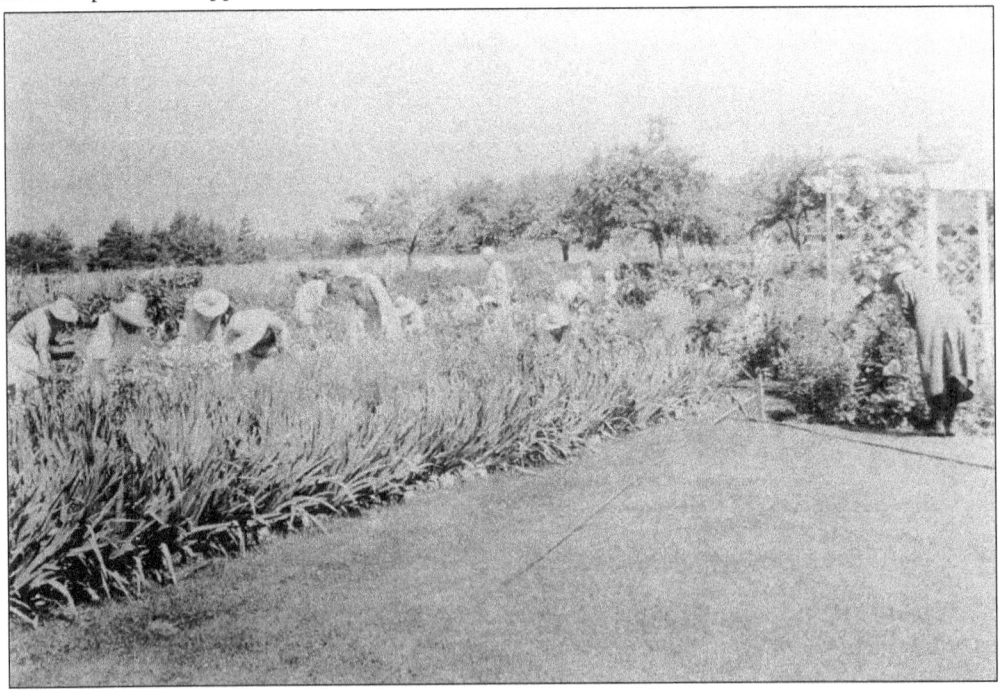

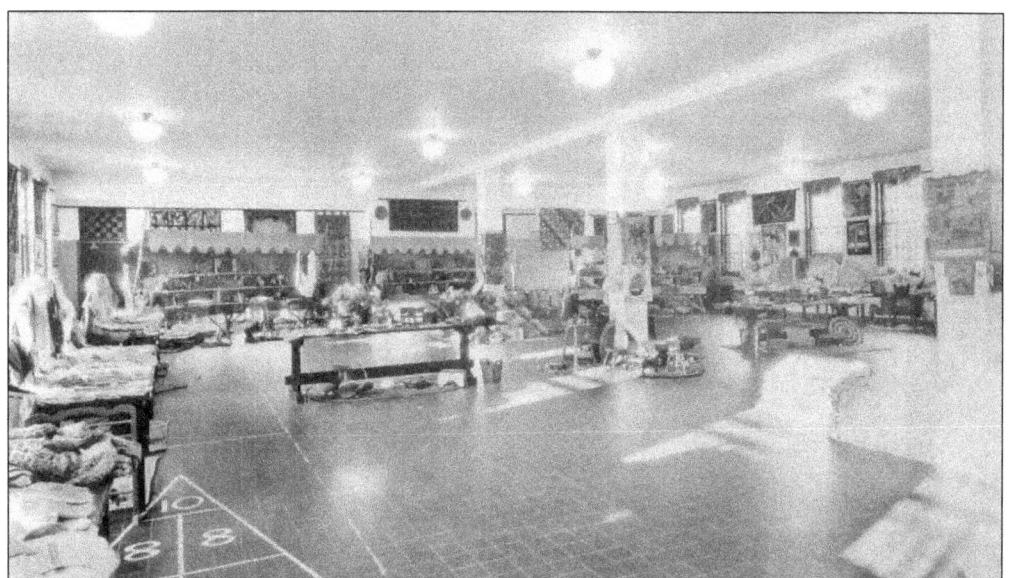

One of the first occupational therapy exhibits and sales at Pilgrim State Hospital is seen here. This fair was held in one of the dining halls and was open to staff and patients. Rugs are proudly displayed from the picture rails around the room. At center, a handful of milking stools await sale.

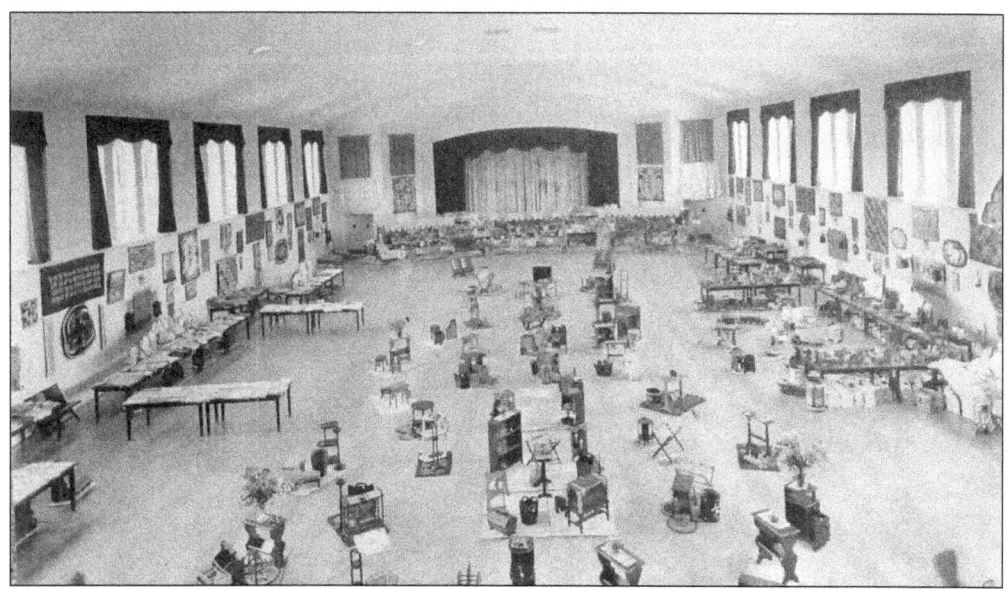

This photograph was taken just a few years after the one above, when construction was completed on the assembly hall at Pilgrim State Hospital. An even more extensive assortment of crafts can be seen at this exhibit. Most notably, there was a surge in the production of furniture. Close inspection reveals that a considerable amount of aptitude was necessary to produce items with such character.

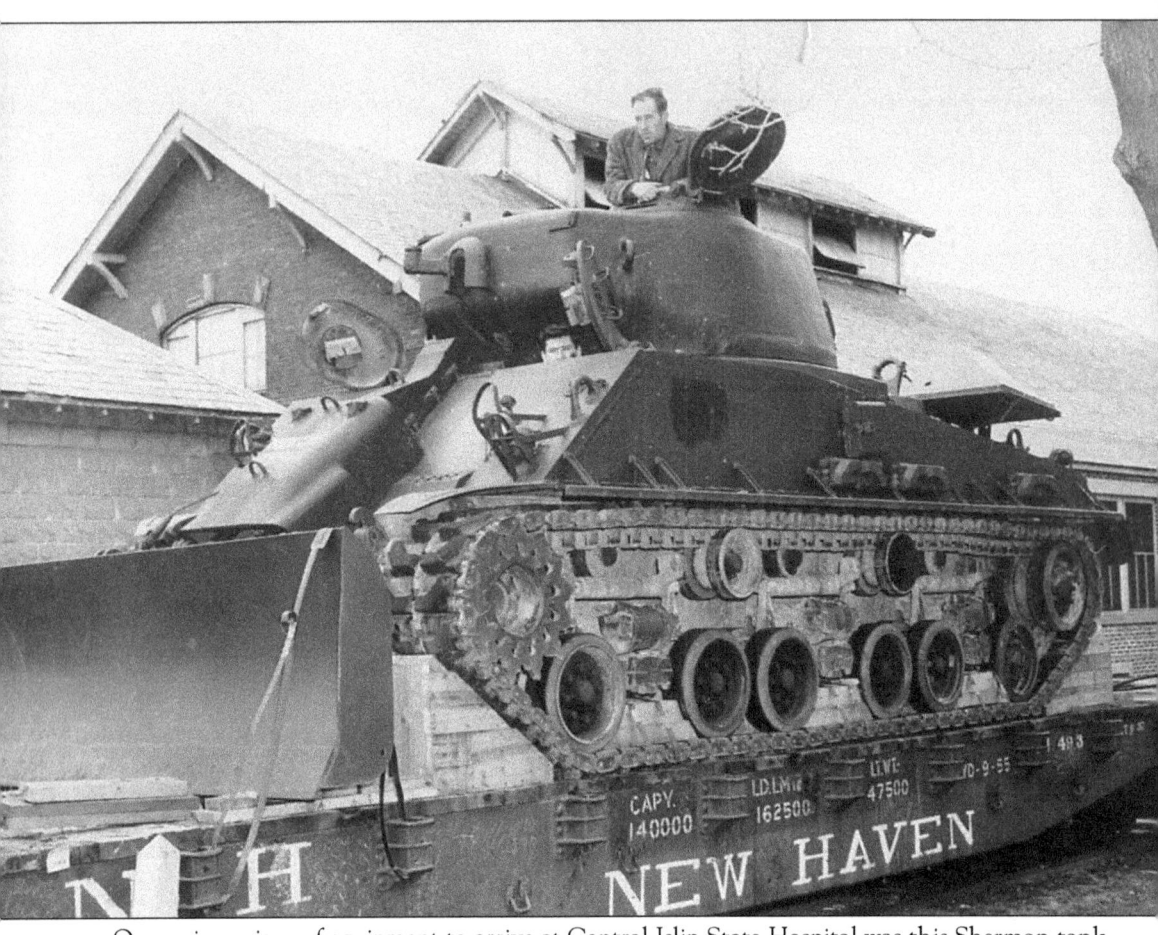

One unique piece of equipment to arrive at Central Islip State Hospital was this Sherman tank decommissioned by the War Department. One of only 50 out of 40,000 Sherman tanks built with a plow attached, it was used by the Army for construction projects. The tank, however, was not delivered with the intention of being deployed against enemy troops. It was retrofitted with the intent of serving as a means of moving train cars and coal, which the power plant used as a fuel source. Here, the tank arrives via rail at the south colony power plant still strapped to the train car. Maintenance staff are already taking a look at their newly acquired machine. The tank was decommissioned and buried at a remote location on the hospital property in 1960. In 1981, word got out to a tank museum about this tank and where it was buried. The tank was excavated and restored and is currently in possession of the American Armored Foundation.

Curtains, bed linens, and clothing, among many other articles, were almost all produced on site. Seen here in the 1890s at Kings Park State Hospital, a woman pedals a manual sewing machine. Other women sew in their rocking chairs on a spring day. (Courtesy of the Kings Park Heritage Museum.)

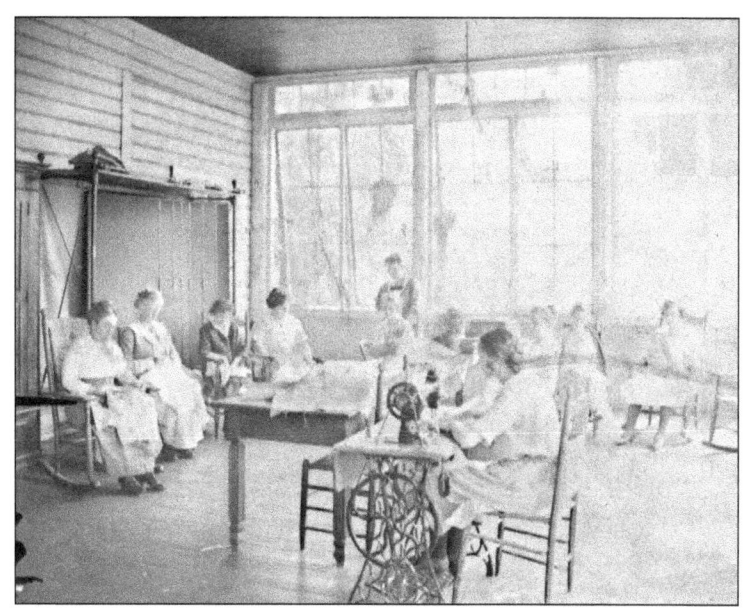

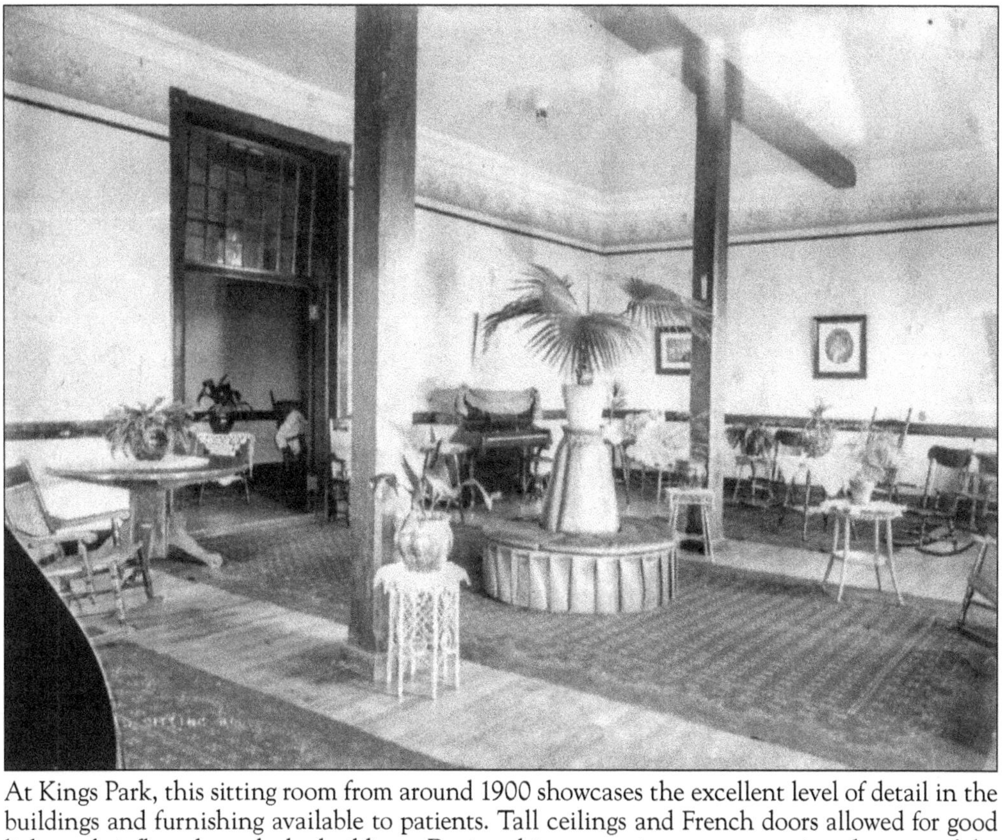

At Kings Park, this sitting room from around 1900 showcases the excellent level of detail in the buildings and furnishing available to patients. Tall ceilings and French doors allowed for good light and airflow through the buildings. During this era, environment was viewed as one of the most critical influences on effective treatment. (Courtesy of the Kings Park Heritage Museum.)

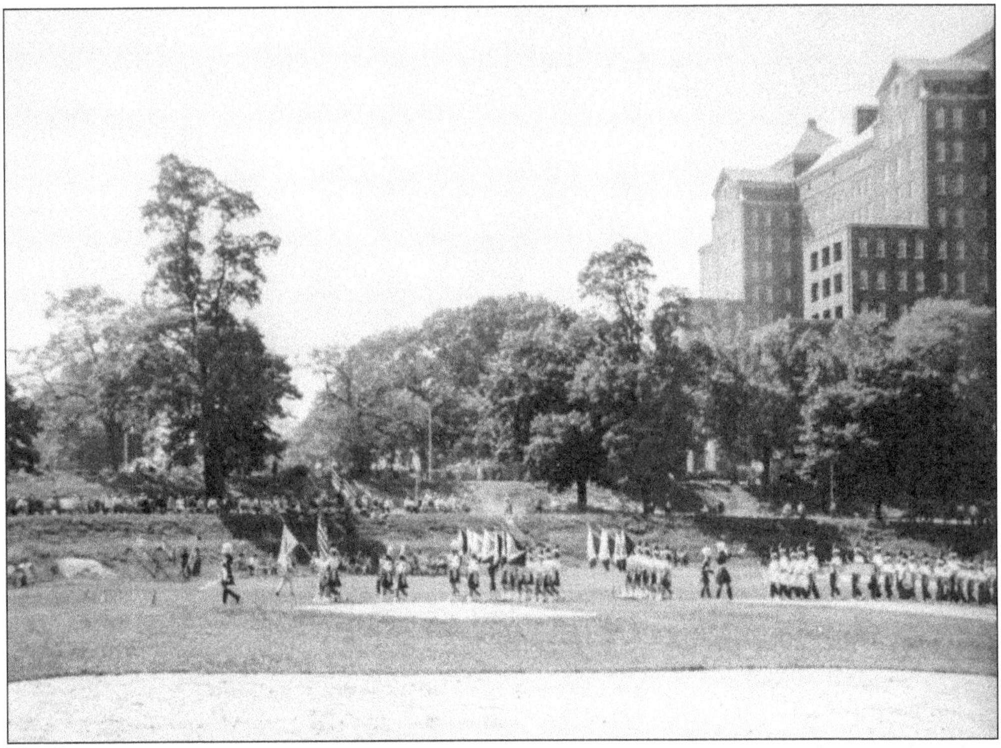

In the earlier part of the 20th century, Kings Park was referred to by many as a botanical garden. The hospital was renowned for its green thumb, manicured grounds, and view of Long Island Sound. Everyone wished to enjoy festivities outside. Here, in a 1940s image captured at Kings Park, the marching band leads off an annual field day of games.

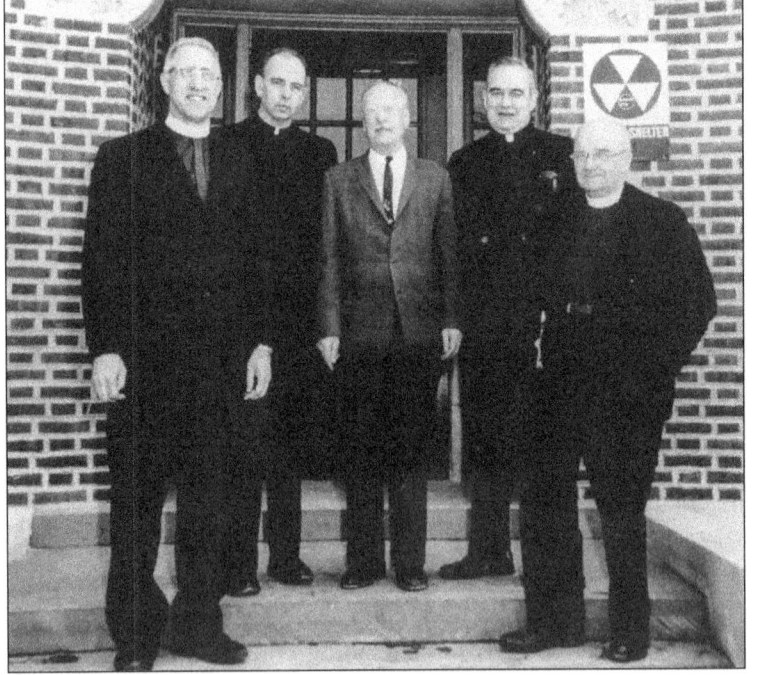

Spiritual guidance and connection have long been important in the lives of people suffering mental affliction. In recent years, spirituality has gained a more respected seat at the table of mental health care. At Pilgrim in the 1960s, this group of chaplains employed by the hospital pose outside a staff dormitory.

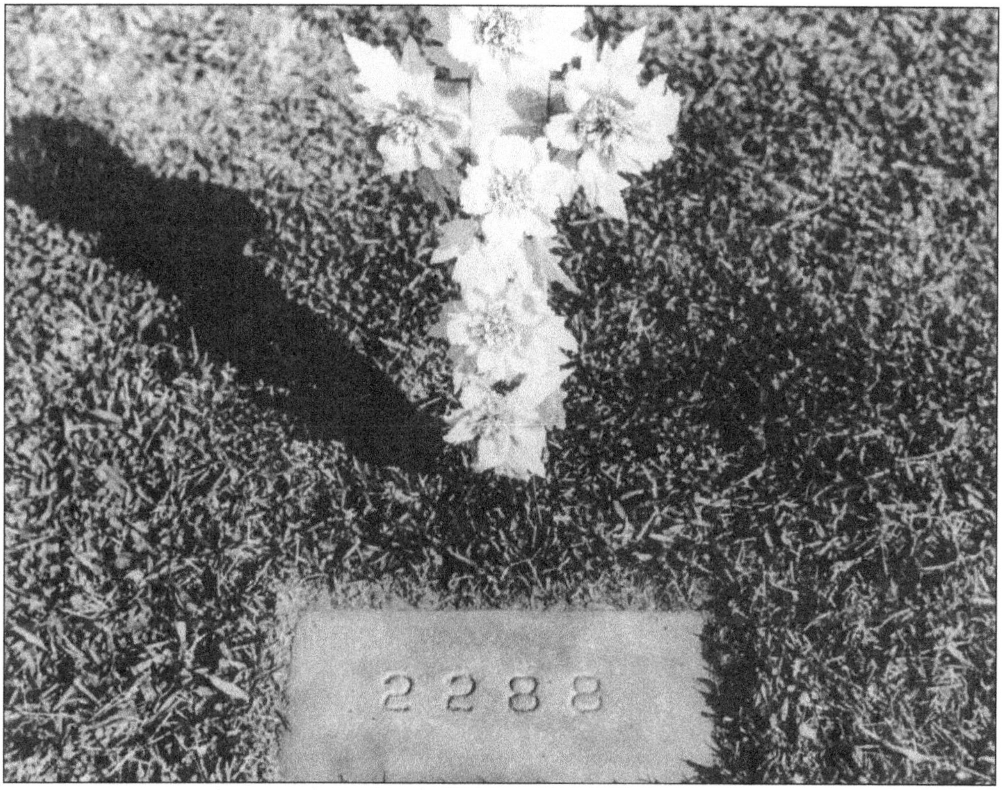

For many patients who passed on, no relatives were willing to provide burial or attend services. Each state hospital had its own cemeteries for patients and staff. In order to provide anonymity, gravestones were marked with numbers and accompanied by a cross or star to denote religious faith. A book of records was kept, with names corresponding to each numbered stone. Funeral services were held on the grounds and were often attended by staff and fellow patients who had befriended a person during their hospitalization. Although only a fraction of the Long Island state hospitals are left intact, their cemeteries remain as a reminder of the lives that once filled the institutions.

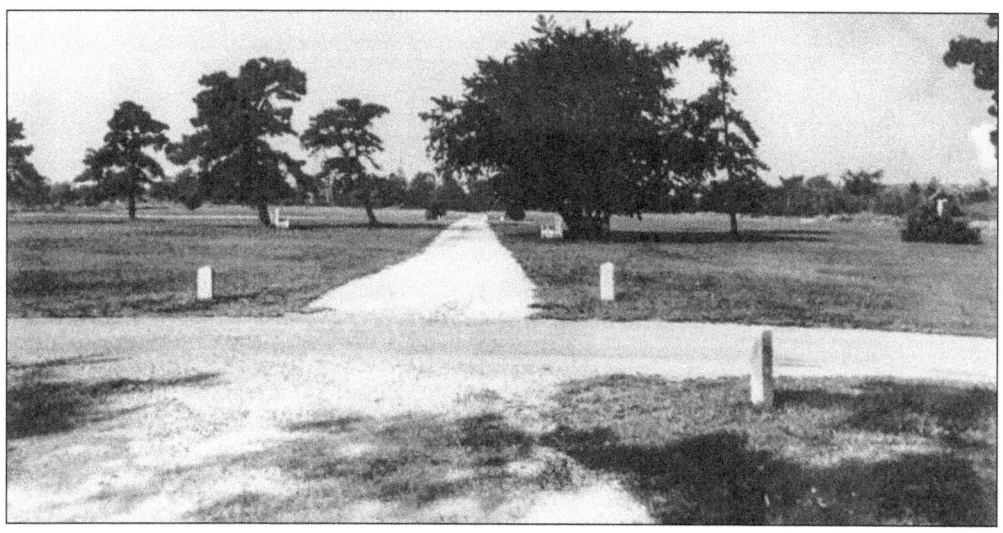

Visit us at
arcadiapublishing.com

www.ingramcontent.com/pod-product-compliance
Lightning Source LLC
Chambersburg PA
CBHW060937170426
43194CB00027B/2985